I love Driven MEN!

David Dream On!

Critical Acclaim for Surviving Cancerland

"Kathleen's story is powerful, honest, and eye-opening. She asks readers to go a bit beyond where some might feel comfortable, but if you are willing, the reward is the story of a profound healing journey. Kathleen tells us, 'My crisis increased my intuition, which in turn saved my life.' Thank you, Kathleen. Miracles and angels are a part of our lives, so anticipate them and tune in through your quiet mind."

— Dr. Bernie Siegel, M.D., author, radio host, inspirational speaker

"Kat is one of the pioneering precognitive dreamers from the Breast Cancer Warning Dreams Research Project. Her amazing stories of dream guides appearing in magical pop-up windows with wise advice for her healing journey can inspire us all to find the guidance that we need during challenging times in our own lives."

— Larry Burk, MD, CEHP, President of Healing Imager, PC, author of *Let Magic Happen: Adventures in Healing with a Holistic Radiologist*

"I often see people who are going through or have just finished cancer treatment because I do their reconstructive surgery, but I never learn the details of their everyday lives. As physicians, we don't know what it is to undergo treatment or how important it is for people to share this experience. Surviving Cancerland can be used as a reference book and is an education for both doctors and laypeople that is positive, not depressing, in its factual account."

— Dr. Helen S. Colen, MD, FACS, PC,
Clinical Associate Professor of Plastic Surgery,
Department of Surgery, NYU Medical Center, NY

"*Armed with an incisive wit, Ms. O'Keefe-Kanavos puts forward her experience as a cancer survivor. Drawing on scientific literature and reviews, she tackles the intellectual aspect of the medical world from the perspective of her personal intuition as a patient. She presents the amazing power of the inner soul and the importance of trusting intuition when facing any diagnosis and treatment. Kathleen steps outside the traditional box to make a persuasive and passionate case for combining medical and spiritual healing and for trusting the God-given gift of intuition. Believing that knowledge is power, I intend to translate Ms. O'Keefe-Kanavos' book into Farsi to give access to many other women outside of the U.S. Knowledge of her journey can inspire everyone to empower and educate themselves as they travel along their personal paths.*"

— Farzaneh Kia, Ph.D., Rancho Mirage, Calif.

"Surviving Cancerland *is a unique perspective on crisis. Much of the literature that comes my way is full of frightening statistics and hopeless stories. Ms. Kanavos has written a book with intention and purpose to allay those fears. There are many aspects to consider from spiritual and treatment modalities. The key is to listen to your body (intuitively) even if the medical community tells you something different. I found this book empowering, positive, and filled with hope and alternatives. I highly recommend it to anyone going through a health trauma.*"

— Nancy Curtin Shea, RN, triple negative breast cancer patient undergoing treatment

"Surviving Cancerland *is a real and revealing account of a woman's struggle through her healing battle with cancer. The book is riveting and witty. Even in the darkest moments, Kathleen manages to find humor and power to advocate for herself, using both her spiritual guides and medical science. Chronicling a person's successful journey to the other side of cancer, this is a great primer for people dealing with this devastating disease.*"

— Suzanne Strisower, MA, PPC, author, coach, and radio show host
www.AwakenToYourLifePurpose.com

"I constantly speak with people who are in the middle of a health crisis. I've heard the stories of those who relied on traditional diagnosis and the stories of those who listened to an internal voice that stated something was amiss. I experienced a knowing from this dialogue. When I listen to this voice, I reap the benefits. When I ignore it, I reap the repercussions. Kathleen's book is a great resource for anyone experiencing this voice or knowing and as a personal story of someone who is living this gift."

— Karen Mayfield, Msc.CC., author, speaker,
founder of Wake Up Women

Kathleen O'Keefe-Kanavos has written a beautiful book describing how important it was for her to listen to her spirit guides and deeply honor her own sense of what her body needed as she moved through the journey of breast cancer diagnosis and treatment. For those about to experience chemotherapy and radiation, Kathleen's humorous and insightful account will help prepare them emotionally, mentally, and spiritually. For people facing cancer, and for their friends and loved ones, this book will inspire and elevate the spirit to better cope with the unknown."

—Neil Nathan, MD, Gordon Medical Associates, Santa Rosa, Calif.,
author of On Hope and Healing: For Those Who Have Fallen
Through the Medical Cracks

SURVIVING CANCERLAND

Intuitive Aspects of Healing

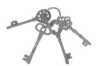

Kathleen O'Keefe-Kanavos

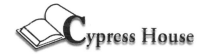

SURVIVING CANCERLAND
Intuitive Aspects of Healing

Cypress House
155 Cypress Street
Fort Bragg, CA 95437
(800) 773-7782
www.cypresshouse.com

Book and Cover Design by Michael Brechner/Cypress House

Front cover illustration © iStockphoto.com/Ann_Mei
Alice in Wonderland figure by John Tenniel (1820–1914)
Drink Me bottle © iStockphoto.com/AnthiaCumming

PUBLISHER'S CATALOGING-IN-PUBLICATION DATA

O'Keefe-Kanavos, Kathleen.
Surviving cancerland : intuitive aspects of healing / Kathleen O'Keefe-Kanavos. -- 1st ed. -- Fort Bragg, CA : Cypress House, c2014.

p. ; cm.

ISBN: 978-1-879384-96-5

Summary: The author's account of how she learned to stand in her power and speak her truth during a life crisis by connecting with her physician-within through dreams, meditations, and prayer. Believing in her intuition, Kathleen used it to self-advocate a course of cancer treatment in her healing process, never forgetting that the patient must make the final decisions.--Publisher.

1. Breast--Cancer--Patients--United States--Biography. 2. Cancer--Patients--United States--Biography. 3. Breast--Cancer--Treatment. 4. Breast--Cancer--Alternative treatment. 5. Cancer--Treatment. 6. Cancer--Alternative treatment. 7. Mind and body therapies. 8. Self-care, Health. 9. Self-help techniques. 10. Intuition. 11. Dreams. 12. Spirituality. I. Title.

RC270.8 .O44 2014	2013947212
616.99/406--dc23	1401

PRINTED IN THE USA
2 4 6 8 9 7 5 3 1

*I dedicate this book to all who have been
involved in the fight against cancer;
those who have won; those still in conflict; and
those who have fallen in battle.*

And to my husband, Peter Kanavos, the love of my life.

Contents

✸

PREFACE

Sometimes you don't know what you are made of until you start to fall apart and your best parts pop out and hold you together. You are made up of so much more than id, ego, and superego. Often, bad things happen to good people. That's life. But you don't have to be a victim of circumstances. Listening to your inner guidance can save you from being a victim at all.

I embarked on a journey similar to *Alice's Adventures in Wonderland* when I fell down the rabbit hole of Cancerland. As a child I had been encouraged to suppress my intuitive gifts: hearing voices, playing with imaginary friends, and drawing auras. These were unacceptable in school and church. I locked my intuitions away in the depths of my mind, but when my life was threatened by misdiagnosis and hospital policy, my guides blew off the doors of their cell and flew to my rescue. Rather than be a victim of circumstance, I self-advocated and became an active participant in my race for life.

My guides led me through my tunnel of crisis and out the other side. Illness drove a bigger story of survival against all odds, while locked in a relationship triangle between my husband and crisis. Who would emerge the victor? I embraced my intuition. Carefully, I built a bridge that, under constant construction, stretched between conventional and metaphysical healing. Beyond it manifested new exits and entrances on the road through Cancerland, to a complete healing of mind, body, and spirit.

Surviving Cancerland provides multiple explanations for the way things are in the physical, spiritual, psychic, and dream worlds of health and emotional trauma and covers all aspects of humanity's complexities and individualism during the process of healing.

Crisis is humbling and comes in many forms, such as a life-threatening illness, a lifestyle change, divorce, death, financial downturn, or all of the above. Crisis is guaranteed to knock you down with its series of catastrophes, often with no end in sight. Your intuition, which is defined as "instinctively knowing without conscious reasoning," can play a crucial part in survival.

I'm writing this book to present an alternative to ignoring your intuition in favor of science or ignoring science in favor of intuition. Why limit yourself to one when you can use both to your advantage?

I've learned that the best way to survive any crisis is to mix intuitional and scientific information, then crosscheck them against each other for answers that are indisputably correct. Listen, then verify. Believe, but validate. By respecting both modalities, you double your chances of finding the correct answer.

It's time to stop ignoring ourselves and discover our voices. Every challenge you overcome creates a new part of your inner voice or personality. To effectively battle crisis, you must marshal your inner "selves" and work with them toward the goal of survival by using everything available. By searching within yourself through dreams, meditation, and prayer, you will find your own set of answers to any challenge.

When faced with crisis many of us are engulfed by fear of the unknown. It was the same for me. When my intuitive suspicion of breast cancer was medically confirmed, I considered suicide as a means of freeing myself from a painful uncertainty. I wanted to avoid the gruesome death suffered by my mother sixteen months earlier. Before I had time to fully grieve for her, I was already grieving for myself. Unfortunately, I, like many of us, had forgotten that I was armed with lessons learned throughout life. Our inner selves are our links to these lessons. We must become reunited with them in our goal to survive.

Everyone battling any life-threatening crisis has his or her own set of questions concerning treatment and survival; however, questions concerning intuition often go unanswered by the medical field, which uses conventional approaches. *Surviving Cancerland* answers those questions.

Spiritual guides, angels, intuition, gut instincts, call them what you will, society gives hearing voices and believing dreams a bad rap. Just ask Joan of Arc. Her voices were a two-edged sword that led her to victory in battle and then to the stake as an alleged witch. Despite what society may perpetuate about dreams, they saved my life. Without their intervention, I believe I'd be dead, and this book would never have been written.

In *Send Me Your Guardian Angel* by Father Alessio Parente, O.F.M. Cap., about the life of Padre Pio, the padre's guardian angel first appeared to him when he was still a boy. "He took the semblance of another child and made himself visible only to me." Later, Padre Pio called his guardian angel/spiritual guide "the companion of my infancy." This could describe my invisible childhood friend, Gee-Gee, who later became a full spiritual guide.

I've learned many important things while fighting for my survival these past ten years:

* You get nowhere standing on the sidelines of the game of Life and Death with crossed fingers waiting for someone else to take action for you.

* Life is not a spectator sport. You are responsible for yourself, so play.

* Your inner self uses signs and symbols that include and go beyond dreams to communicate with you, especially during any crisis such as divorce, financial problems, and health issues.

* No matter how confusing they may seem, your dreams are always telling you something.

* Synchronicities can be validations of intuitive knowings, actions, and guidance.

* Listen to your fears, but don't let them rule your life; let them guide you to action.

* Be a squeaky wheel. Don't take no for an answer. Don't settle for less. And don't be dismissed. Hoping someone else will make

the right decisions for you when you are in crisis is a half-plan, missing a vital component and your biggest resource: YOU.

* Take care of your Spirit and it will take care of you.

* You can apply the empowering information in this book to all of your life challenges.

For many reasons, I never intended to write a book using my diaries. First, life is too short to wallow in nostalgia, and second, I'm a very private person. My diaries are *extremely* personal, and are filled with sexually intimate and psychic phenomena. Yet, five years later, when faced with recurrence and searching for forgotten information often scribbled on cash receipts and napkins taped or glued to notebook pages, I realized I must share this extraordinary journey of self-advocacy. Those scribbled notes became lifesaving lessons based not on blind faith but on the ability to trust knowledge imparted from other, unseen dimensions of existence. I refused to be a victim to circumstance.

Surviving Cancerland spotlights an unmet need and illuminates an aspect of crisis that has remained in the dark: the spiritual realm of healing from the patient's point of view and how you can use inner thoughts, voices, dreams, and nightmares for navigation and to provide humor for healing.

Your Key Ring of Life is loaded with keys of all sort and sizes; they fit many doors known as Life Lessons. Big skeleton keys fit many locks, while smaller keys fit tiny doors of immense importance and opportunity. Sorting through them can be confusing and time consuming. I've done the work for you.

At the end of each chapter you'll find Survival Keys necessary to open your doors within doors, behind which are Life Lessons to help you find your Intuitive Gifts to survive. Once you find them, use the steps I've provided to connect with your Inner Guidance. I offer this to everyone now with the tiny, powerful keys of hope and love.

Acknowledgments

I could never have survived this difficult time without the love and devotion of Peter, my husband and best friend. He laughed, cried, partied, and experienced sympathy pains with me throughout my ordeal.

I wish to thank all the brave people who shared their deeply personal experiences while walking down the twisted, scary road of cancer, wondering where it would end, if it would end, and most frightening... how it would end.

Special thanks to my Boston doctors and medical personnel from the Brigham and Women's Hospital and Dana-Farber Cancer Institute for your help and reassurance.

Thank you to Susan A. Schwartz and Josephine Salata for all your editorial help. And a special thanks to all the friends who read my manuscript many times and shared their two cents, which made me wealthy in words.

I could never have interpreted some of my more difficult dreams without the help of Ursula Martins, and to you, Ursula, I am truly grateful.

Thank you, Petronelle Cook, AKA Margot Arnold, devoted friend, mentor, and author who read my many drafts and encouraged me whenever I had doubts about my book, writing skills, and psychic gifts.

Special thanks to all the people who read and wrote comments on the book, including Suzanne Strisower, Mary Cate O'Malley, and Dr. Farzaneh Kia, who went beyond the call of duty by offering to translate *Surviving Cancerland* so Middle Eastern women could read it.

And finally, thank you, Mom, for your constant loving help from "the other side."

My book practically wrote itself with the help of my spiritual guides. Thank you, guides, for all your support, but above all, I thank God for sending me those protective spiritual guiding lights. Miracles are indeed still a part of our daily lives.

Surviving
Cancerland

Part 1

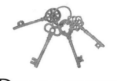

Discovery

Chapter 1
Discovery and "Voices"

What a wonderful life I've had!
I only wish I'd realized it sooner.
— Colette (1873–1954)

♥ *Affirmation:* Loving myself heals my life.

A deadly storm brews as I recline against Peter's chest during our nightly bath ritual. As I massage him, he lathers my body with fragrant bubbles. The tranquility within our bathroom offsets a Cape Cod nor'easter building over the bay. Romantic candles and music make the squall appear benign through the large skylight. Halloween had passed weeks ago, yet the sky remains in rich costume. Black velvet clouds fondle a full moon, while angry winds rattle windows and howl like hungry wolves. I adjust myself in the bath to better view the macabre performance of moonlight's struggle against darkness and wait for the storm to pass. The serenity of our bathtub snuggle session is shattered by a life-altering question that forebodes a deadlier squall building within our lives.

"Kathy, what's this hard spot?" Peter asks over my shoulder as he gently caresses my breasts with soapy hands.

My hand absentmindedly follows his to what feels like a pea beneath my skin. His voice is suddenly replaced by the memory of a dream I had had after a recent mammogram, and another voice — an inner one — declares, "*Get to a doctor, now!*" I've never been sick in my life, to speak of, and illness is not a concern, yet a storm has just invaded our lives.

3

Three days later, I'm at an appointment with my gynecologist and general practitioner, Dr. Dennis Wagner, who resembles the late Gary Cooper in physique and demeanor. Each time Dr. Wagner enters the examining room, the theme song from *High Noon* plays in my head. I expect a Colt .44 on his hip rather than a stethoscope around his neck. "I can't feel anything on or around your breast, Kathy."

"Perhaps it's easier to feel during my menstrual cycle," I reply, contorted with my arm over my head. He shakes his head as he manipulates the area again. I'm torn between relief and concern. Is nothing really there? Has he missed it, or are the voices of alarm in my head just residual anxiety from Mom's recent death from colon cancer? But Peter felt it, too.

"You had a blood test and mammogram less than six months ago and everything was fine," Dr. Wagner says. He helps me up and shows me a copy of the report. "I think what you felt was just a fibrous tumor that is sensitive to your menstrual cycle. Let's keep an eye on it. Come back in six months, and we'll check it again," he concludes with a reassuring smile, snapping my chart shut. We speak a few minutes longer about how little cancer there is in my family history, and my mind wanders back to a day, not that long ago, now feeling like a lifetime, to a heartbreaking "cancer talk" with Mom.

Her gurney was pushed against the corridor wall as she waited for an ultrasound to see the extent of her metastasis. Our final mother-daughter conversation began, "Breast cancer doesn't run in our family, but now colon cancer does. You must get a colonoscopy and be vigilant of symptoms." She smiled through eyes filled with sadness, pain, and love. Was her grief unwarranted guilt at having brought this dreaded disease into our previously cancer-free family? That would prove to be the second saddest day of my life. The first would be her death, just two days later.

"You're only forty-four — too young for cancer, you know." Dr. Wagner's words shock me back to the present. If he isn't worried about this invisible hard spot, why am I? After all, he's the doctor, right? I dress and head for home, worry free.

But the voices from my bath refuse to be silent. They are in my every nagging thought and daydream. "*Go back to your doctor,*" they say. I have a choice: let these voices drive me crazy or listen so they'll shut up. Three days later, I return to Dr. Wagner who gives me another mammogram and blood test. "Go home. I'll call you with the results," he promises.

Almost one more month passes, and on my forty-fourth birthday I receive two questionable gifts: another cancer-free mammogram and *Happy Birthday* sung solo to me over the telephone by my father. It must be as difficult for him to sing it as it is for me to hear it. There is no high-pitched female voice to chime in on a different note or end with "and many more," punctuated by a heartfelt laugh. Well, my healthy mammogram proves I'll have more birthdays — unfortunately without Mom. A blessing and a torment all tied in a pink ribbon of lonely lyrics.

That night's strange dream would send me scurrying back to Dr. Wagner. Enjoying my dream, it suddenly stops, much like what happens when a computer screen freezes, and a pop-up window appears, also similar to that of a computer. My spiritual guide/guardian angel, in the brown robe, rope belt, and leather sandals of a monk, steps through the window and says, "*Come with me. We have something to tell you.*" I obediently follow him into a room I call the Room Between Realms, a place that is neither of the living nor the dead, yet both can visit to share information. It is a parallel universe of consciousness. A guide takes my hand, places it on my right breast, and says, "*You have cancer right here. Feel it? Go back to your doctor tomorrow. Don't wait for an appointment.*" I start to cry and tell him that the doctors won't listen to me now any more than before. "They just keep giving me the same tests over and over. You help me."

My guide reaches into the pocket of his robe and hands me a tiny white feather, no bigger than one that might escape a pillow and glide to a bedroom floor. "*Use this feather as a sword to fence with in your verbal battles with the doctors and you will win against scientific facts. You need exploratory surgery. If you present your case to the doctors as though you were an attorney standing before an incredulous judge who dislikes you, you will win,*" he says, then turns and walks out of my dream. I'm outside the Room Between Realms as the window disappears. My previous dream starts where it left off. Time had stood still.

I've reached a crossroads: Do I believe the doctors or the voices? And how do I explain to the one I decide not to believe, my decision to believe the other?

The truth is, most people do not consider hearing voices a good thing, yet I'm being pushed into action by unseen forces, making me feel out of control, like a victim of circumstance. It appears I have two choices: ignore these voices and tell them to go away, or use them to guide me in a showdown with my doctor. Should I tell him about the voices? I know how doctors feel about voices, and it's about as good as teachers feel about them, as I learned in kindergarten.

"Kathy is coloring people funny colors outside the lines," my teacher explained to my parents at the emergency conference she had scheduled. My mother reacted as any concerned parent would have. She took me to an ophthalmologist. He determined that my eyes were fine but that I was in need of attention. His parting words to me were "You color things correctly from now on and stay inside the lines. Stop worrying your mother."

That was the first time I realized that the rest of the world, including doctors with their fancy equipment, couldn't see what I was seeing: *auras*, the colorful electromagnetic fields that surround each thing in the universe. Explaining my colorings to them would be like describing a shrub covered in pink flowers to someone with red-green colorblindness. Their normal reaction: "What flowers? Check her eyes! There's something *wrong* with her."

History repeats itself now as my doctor becomes alarmed at my latest request. The look of horror on his face says it all. "You want exploratory surgery? I can't take something out that isn't there. An operation is a serious decision, and in your case unfounded and unnecessary." He is upset. So am I, but for a different reason. His concern is that I've overreacted to an "invisible spot." Mine is that I haven't reacted *enough* to this damned spot.

As a doctor, he is armed with indisputable medical evidence: three mammograms, blood tests, and physical exams that all point to perfect health. I'm armed only with an angel feather from a dream. I dig into my mental chest, pull out the tiny feather, and imagine pointing it at him. His defense seems logically indisputable, yet I plead my case like a lawyer to convince him to do what I want and not play a "wait and see" game. Six months may be too late. But since I'm the patient and he the doctor, I am at his mercy. *I'm taking a giant leap of faith here, so "voices," don't let me down!* I silently pray, while mentally pinching my feather between my fingers. Then I turn to face my medical opponent, whom I must turn into an ally.

 ## Survival Keys

* Self-advocate. Never be afraid to self-advocate for your life or beliefs.

* Challenge the status quo. If it were never challenged, the world would still be flat.

* Stand in your power and speak your truth.

Chapter 2

POLICY VS. PEOPLE

A dream that is not interpreted is like a letter that is not read.
— The Talmud

♥ *Affirmation:* I choose to see difficulties in life as
intentions to make me better, not bitter.

"I've had time to think things over. I want this questionable hard spot out as soon as possible," I explain to Dr. Wagner. "It doesn't feel right, and you know me — I'm not the type of person who keeps showing up on your doorstep begging to be operated on, nor am I a hypochondriac. I have to go with my instincts."

Calm, I maintain eye contact so my doctor can see that I am resolute in my decision.

"Kathy, I can't just cut you open because you want me to. It's against hospital policy and my policy. There are dangers, such as infection and anesthesia complications."

I stand my ground and repeat myself.

He studies me and then says, "Okay."

Did he just say okay? I feel so relieved I want to jump off the table and hug him. I've done it! I fenced with a feather and won, despite opposing medical evaluations, tests, facts, and hospital policy. But my victory is bittersweet. I'm about to be cut open and explored. I put my feather away and gasp.

His fingertips gently knead the area below my right armpit at the eleven o'clock position. "I can feel something here, but I think it's nothing important or it would have shown up on the tests. I'll cut down

8

over this spot. It doesn't feel at all like cancer, which doesn't have smooth edges like this." I look at him with pleading eyes that beg him to change his mind and perform the operation. "But if you insist, I'll take it out. First let's see if it's just another cyst."

He inserts a needle into the area and draws back the plunger. The syringe fills with blood; excruciating pain follows. This is not normal. I'd had cysts aspirated before and drawing the tea-colored fluid had been painless and bloodless. Afraid the needle will break off in my breast, I grip the side of the table to steady myself during the agony. He looks concerned, helps me sit up, and leaves the room.

I pull the torn, bloodied paper gown across my chest as if protecting myself from a new thought: *If that damned spot is cancerous, are the cells now loose in my bloodstream?* I remember having read that, during operations, cancerous areas accelerate their growth from air and blood transfer. Is this outdated information, or did he just shove a stick into a hornet's nest? In my panic, beads of perspiration build on my scalp as my mouth becomes dry.

Returning to the room, Dr. Wagner says, "The earliest date available to operate is a few days after the New Year. It will be day surgery, so you won't stay in the hospital overnight."

This is a complete turnaround from his previous reaction to my *unfounded* request. Was it the blood, the pain, or was he hearing voices, too? I try to read his expression but get that Gary Cooper poker face. My surgery is scheduled at Boston's Brigham and Women's Hospital, just one week away.

"Who will perform the surgery?" I ask while I button my shirt. The question takes on an unusual importance as it echoes through my mind.

"I will. You won't need an oncologist there. You don't have cancer."

I ponder this statement as I slip the last button through its buttonhole. Am I making a mistake by not pushing for an oncologist at the procedure? I hope not, but what can I do? If I push, he might change his mind. I had just been victorious in self-advocating with a feather. I don't want to follow that with defeat. And where will I find an oncologist or another doctor at the last minute without a recommendation?

Happy Holidays!

What a nightmare. Where's my feather? I'm leaving.

Since all this occurred, rest had not come easily at night. I love to dream. My dreams are so detailed they could win Academy Awards. But lately they had become nightmares.

Here is one. As I sleep, another pop-up window to the other side appears — a doorway to the Room Between Realms, a meeting place for the living and the dead that I've visited many times. I name this dream "The Pop-up."

I walk down a narrow hallway. Discarded clothing is strewn on chairs. Through a door, I see Mom get out of her bed. She smiles, waves, and holds out her hands in greeting as she walks barefoot toward me. I step through the door, grab her hands, pull myself to her, hug her tightly, and say, "I miss you so much, Mom."

"I miss you, too," she answers calmly. She appears to have accepted her death better than I. The experience is so real I can feel the moles on her back through her nightgown, the same one she'd worn the night she died. Her special individual smell that overrides perfume fills me with memories. I know that we are in the realm between realms and that Mom might disappear at any moment. This spot is only a temporary meeting place. "You are going to be just fine," Mom says, then slowly dissipates into thin air as I'm left hugging myself. Next, the dream window disappears, and I'm back in my original dream, right where I'd left off. I wake up crying. Had I been given a reassuring visit from Mom? If so, why am I so sad? And how am I going to be "just fine?"

Interpretation: This is a lucid, spirit-guided, prophetic dream containing dualities. I'm aware of dreaming while sleeping. It is not a dream about my mother. I'm actually visiting with her in an area between realms. This is the first time I am seeing and speaking with Mom since her death, yet she knows what I'm experiencing and had come to comfort and reassure me.

Was this divination? Did I dare hope? Either way it was a wonderful Christmas gift because I spent time with Mom, if only a few seconds.

This was not the first time I had stepped through a pop-up to speak with the dead. Shortly before Peter and I married, Jack, a twenty-eight-year-old family member, died. His girlfriend found him seated on the couch in front of the TV with his legs crossed and a doughnut on his chest. The police had sealed the apartment before we got there, and I watched as a shiny black bag on a mortuary stretcher was wheeled away.

That night a dream pop-up appeared. Jack stepped through it and walked up to me. "I always thought I would go out in a blaze, but I just fell asleep," he said. Dressed in shorts, his favorite black leather jacket, and black-and-white sneakers, Jack repeated himself, laughed, and walked back through the pop-up, which closed behind him. My original dream continued.

The next morning, I told Peter about my dream and Jack's comment. Peter said he would be very surprised if Jack had just fallen asleep and died.

Two weeks later the coroner's report stated that Jack's body had shut down, and his death was ruled natural. When Jack's clothes were returned from the coroner's office, they were the same ones he had worn in the dream. A month later, Jack appeared to me again, in his apartment, accompanied by a black-and-white cat. At first I didn't know him because he constantly switched in and out of different bodies. Eventually I recognized him by his eyes.

"Jack, why are you still here, and where's your body?"

"I didn't respect it, so I must borrow one to speak with you," he replied. A spirit guide in a brown hooded robe appeared next to him as the cat sniffed potted plants.

"What can I do for you, Jack?" I asked as much to the guide as to him.

"I need for my family to understand me. I was uncommunicative in life and now I can't communicate with them. I have to stay here until they understand me. I feel so alone." He touched my arm, and I recoiled from the overwhelming feeling of emptiness that engulfed me. I woke up yelling. I don't want it written about Jack 200 years from now that he wanders the earth as a restless spirit in haunted houses, but I don't know how to help.

That problem would be solved several nights later when again, in the middle of a peaceful dream, a pop-up occurred and two hooded guides led me into a dimly lit brick room with a large roaring fireplace. I was instructed to sit silently in the center of three empty chairs and listen. All night long, two guides on either side of me discussed every aspect of Jack's life, from the type of birth control he and his girlfriend had used to his hidden gun. I was told to share the information "with those who mattered" and was then led back to my dream.

Much of what I told Jack's friends and family was immediately validated, including the cat. His mother said I had described a pet that had been dead and forgotten for fifteen years. However, his family discovered a sensitive Jack. This new insight dissolved their guilt and grief, which may have held Jack back from "moving on."

A few nights later I silently spoke to Jack while preparing for sleep. *"Did this help you, Jack? I don't want you stuck in the area between realms."* That last part was said as much to the spirit guides as to him. A voice in my mind answered, *"Jack will be here for ninety days, and then he will be ready."*

"Ready for what?" I wondered in response, but received no answer.

Now, a decade later, I wonder if this was training for my own recent guided dreams. The confidence I gained from those previous dream validations might help me as I decide between believing doctors and medical tests or dreams and voices. If life is a school, then it's a good thing I took copious notes in my strange dream classes over the years. I was about to need them.

With only a few days before surgery, I try to enjoy myself at a fantastic New Year's Eve party in a beautiful, castle-like ocean-side resort. When I made the reservation months ago, I had looked forward to this night. Now I don't want to be here. I'm antsy from anxiety and vacillate between hyperactivity and the inability to move: fight or flight and frozen by fear. I alternately hold my breath and sigh.

"Look, Kathy, let us make plane reservations to Aspen for you. We've rented a big condo to ski for the week. Stop worrying. Everything will be fine," my brother-in-law reassures me while helping himself to caviar from the lavish buffet. He hands me another glass of champagne and waits for my response. Peter and Dayssi join us and try to act nonchalant as they stand beside me. They too await my answer.

"No. If everything turns out well, I'll meet you in Aspen."

Mentally and emotionally I can't make plans to go skiing in the future, because I'm stuck in the present, my frightening and crazy "now." This "now" is the place gurus have attempted to reach for decades, yet I feel I'm held prisoner here against my will. If this is nirvana, it sucks. I'd much rather plan a ski trip, but my mind won't let me move forward or backward — too daunting, too traumatic. Only in my sleep can I move forward and backward between dreams and nightmares. But there is a twist to my predicament. (There always seems to be a twist to my predicaments.)

My dreams and nightmares are opening previously locked doors that hold secrets to my future — spiritual information I need to survive. And my inner voices are the ribbon that binds everything together. Fun must wait while I deal with my frightening "now." As I ponder this new state of unwelcome higher consciousness, I feel the onset of another anxiety attack and gulp down my champagne. How and why is this happening to me?

I am a gentle, mature flower child. Mom said that rather than kill a fly, I would open windows and "invite it out." She was right. I still do. I avoid confrontation. My assertive behavior is puzzling. Where did it come from? Gee-Gee hasn't been around since the fifth grade.

I miss Gee-Gee, my imaginary childhood friend, for the first time in thirty-five years. He had been with me in my crib, and often was the only friend of an army brat and only child. With Gee-Gee, I never had to guess, read dream symbols, or color inside the lines. He always told it like it was. And for a small, dark-haired, eight-year-old imaginary boy, he was a master at escape. Gee-Gee, *where are you now?* I silently ask my fifth glass of champagne, as if he might be hiding in the bubbles. "Can you still hear me? I think I need another escape plan," I sigh.

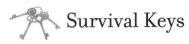 Survival Keys

* Self-advocate with self-respect. This is the sister to "Stand in your power and speak your truth" and a key to success in all areas of life.

* Dare to feel. As Jack's touch demonstrated, even in death, the inability to emotionally feel because of a lack of self is far worse than pain.

* Communicate. Communication is the antidote to emptiness and despair.

Chapter 3

Haunted House or Head Case?

When one door of happiness closes, another opens;
but which has opened? Often we look so long at the
closed door that we do not see the one for us.
— Helen Keller (1880–1968)

♥ *Affirmation:* The more grateful I am, the more reasons
I find to be grateful.

Without any warning, my housekeeper quits. She phones with a startling revelation: Someone or something in our house is watching her as she cleans. "You are the sweetest person I know, but I cannot clean your house anymore. It scares me. I'm not coming back."

Perhaps deceased family members, like Mom, are hanging around to give me support, but I decide it's unwise to explain this to a Jehovah's Witness, so I wish her luck and hang up. Helpful dead family members can be two-edged swords.

Now what do I do for a housekeeper? My surgery is this week.

A voice in my mind answers, "*Look in the* Yellow Pages."

"*The phone book? Are you kidding? I need someone with recommendations I can trust,*" I argue.

"*The Yellow Pages,*" the voice repeats. So I do open them, and lo and behold, I find a company — and it rhymes with Ghostbusters — a perfect fit under the circumstances. The owner even quotes me a better price. One door closes, a better one opens. Now I'll return to a clean home after surgery. I can't believe my luck. Everything is falling so neatly into place.

Dr. Wagner schedules a last-minute MRI to guide him during surgery. Why didn't he decide to do that sooner? Well, better late than never. The morning of the MRI is frigid, a typical Cape Cod January day with windows rattling from gale-force winds. This doesn't seem fair. I should be in warm California playing tennis. Well, I'm not. *Life isn't fair, it's real, so deal*, I remind myself.

As I sprint out the door, Peter yells from the car, "Did you get the message from the MRI clinic to wear pants with an elastic waist and warm socks?" I answer him with a midair spin and head back upstairs to my closet. I'm wearing a sweater dress with boots. Do I own a pair of pants with an elastic waistband? I have a pair of cashmere pajamas I could wear in a pinch. Yup, this qualifies as a pinch. The matching bathrobe can be worn as a sweater, too. Who'll know the difference? *I'm late*, I think, as I glance at my watch and run out the door like the White Rabbit in *Alice in Wonderland*.

"Aren't those your pajamas?" Peter asks as we back out of the driveway. *Darn!*

Everything feels so rushed. Hopefully this MRI will show more than my imagination. It occurs to me that I will freak out if it shows a feather.

Despite my cell phone dropping calls, I finally reach the MRI center to warn them that we might be late. Despite this, by the time we arrive, my slot has been given to someone who came early, leaving me a forty-five-minute wait before the next appointment. This is turning out to be one of those days. As we sit in the waiting room, I feel the approach of another anxiety attack.

The nurse escorting me into the processing room instructs me, "Undress only from the waist up since your pants have an elastic waistband." I hope this is a sign that things are looking up. But I've never had an MRI before. Needles are not my friends. And I'm nervous, as a technician, who looks all of thirteen, explains the need for yellow dye to be inserted by IV. Music by Sting plays on the audio system, as I shiver in my "jammie" bottoms.

The MRI room contains a large, white tubular machine with a bottom drawer that slides in and out by remote control. Its surface has two holes like the ones I use to dig at the beach to accommodate my breasts so I could lie on my stomach and tan my back. The technician explains that the Faulkner Hospital scans both breasts simultaneously while other places only do one breast per appointment. "My breasts are here together, so thank you," I joke.

"Let's try the other arm," the technician says, after sticking and digging for my vein again.

"Let's not," I reply, ready to throw up. "Please, call an IV nurse."

The IV nurse arrives with her portable IV bag. "I'm used to emergency patients who are in shock and often dehydrated. I like challenges," she says as she slides the needle into my vein. Not only is she excellent and accommodating, she uses a needle that can be left in place for the pre-surgery blood work later in the day.

Earplugs make the machine's noise bearable. To my relief, rather than an annoying din, it sounds like boat engines and the playful spotted and bottlenose dolphins who "clicked" at Peter and me with their sonar and followed us like puppies on our scuba-diving trips to the Bahamas.

I manage to hold perfectly still during the thirty-minute session by pretending to be back in warm Bahamian waters, while performing the same meditation I practice each night.

On the ride home, I surprise Peter with a decision I had made earlier in the week by returning my engagement ring to him. Peter's mother and her best friend (whom I consider my Jewish mother, I love her that much) had been kind enough to go with me to pick out the ring, but I felt choosing it should have been *our* special event. I know how Princess Diana felt when Prince Charles sent her a tray of gorgeous gems from which to choose her engagement ring — all by herself. Somehow, I felt I had lost my personal power when I accepted my ring in that way, so despite its size, I despise the thing. Now I'm taking the first step in getting that power back by speaking my truth.

"We're strong enough to look at situations in our life and marriage and change what doesn't work," I say to Peter. "We'll be stronger as individuals and as a unit. Maybe when I stop changing you won't want the new me." This is an important conversation. I choose my words carefully.

"I already see the new, stronger you and still love you. Don't reconsider too many things at this time, Bunny," Peter says, using my pet name. With tears in his eyes he reaches for my hand and promises, "We'll pick out rings together, later."

Later, as we walk through the snow-covered gardens with Baby Cakes, our fifteen-year-old cat, I tell Peter about a dream that had been bothering me and that was somewhat responsible for my ring decision.

In the dream, a young secretary in a hospital waiting room holds a clipboard in her hand and tells me the doctors are going to call me. "You have let this go on for way too long and now it has gotten into everything," she says, and then disappears.

Interpretation: The dream is a duality that says I need to heal my inner self and my life. I had allowed things that had bothered me to go on for far too long by being passive. In the physical realm, the dream told me this lump the doctors can't see is much worse than I think, and it's been there far too long.

This dream scares me. God, I hope it's not cancer in my lymph nodes or throughout my body. Well, only time will tell. Maybe one of the doctors I need is a psychiatrist, because I think I'm on the verge of a breakdown.

Peter listens quietly. What can he say? This is a serious time. I've reached a crossroads of my past relationship and my present body. Changes must be made if I am to have a future. Digging this deep is exhausting. I need a nap. As we fall asleep Peter tells me again that he loves me and can feel the emergence of a new, stronger me. Sandwiched between love, his chest at my front and a purring Baby Cakes at my back, I fall asleep. Standing in my power and speaking my truth has given me rest.

We stay overnight in Boston the day before my surgery to have fun and avoid the morning rush hour. I distract myself with my favorite hobby — shopping — and buy a pair of cashmere socks to wear into surgery. I don't like cold feet.

My last pre-surgery meal at Legal Sea Foods feels like a meal on death row. Butterflies of fear crowd my stomach. I try to stay busy in the moment and not dwell on tomorrow, but I know it will soon be here. I chew off an acrylic fingernail.

The prior night had produced another nightmare. Tired of dreaming, I want to sleep without getting frightening messages. I want to awaken refreshed, not anxious with a racing heart and mind. Mostly, I seek sleep to forget, for it's when I awaken that the nightmare seems most real.

I name this dream "Dolphins and Waterspouts."

I walk along a beach with my mother and Jeanne, an instructor at the Virginia Beach Psychic Institute. Storm clouds build on the horizon. Dolphin fins break the surface of turbulent ocean water. I tell Jeanne to get into the water with me and lie on her stomach. "We'll hold on to the sand and point our feet toward the dolphins. They'll place their noses in our arches to keep us from being pulled out to sea." A loud thunderclap to the right draws our attention to a large waterspout. The dolphins leave us and swim toward a group of people closer to three newly formed waterspouts. As the dolphins approach, the waterspouts explode. An aggressive man in the distant group threatens to cut people's throats with a sharpened coat hanger. "Why are you looking at me?" he yells at me. An African American crowd surrounds and contains him.

We leave the beach and enter our high-rise apartment building, which has three lower floors connected by an escalator and a flight of steep stairs that lead to our penthouse. Jeanne runs up and down the escalator to see how fast she can travel between floors, but the stairs are so steep I must climb them on hands and knees. African Americans live next door to us on the left. With much difficulty they get the aggressive man into the apartment. When it is safe we enter our apartment on the right.

Interpretation: This precognitive dream of Divine intervention and health deals with the future, progress, integration, cooperation, recognition of danger, and choices. The storm on the horizon represents the storm and danger brewing in my life. Fortunately, I have divine support from the dolphins that act as spirit guides.

Jeanne is very pleased when I read her this dream. She says I've decided not to die but rather to stay in the earth plane by holding onto the beach while also fighting in the spiritual plane of water. I wonder if this dream full of threes will take on new meaning after tomorrow's surgery.

 ## Survival Keys

* Fearlessly see crisis for what it is. Crisis leaves no belief systems or relationships unchallenged. It shakes your world to its foundations.

* Learn to welcome "baptism by fire." Daily focus shifts from existence to self-preservation, but baptism by fire is cleansing. In its wake new growth emerges.

* Don't tell your Higher Power how big your troubles are—tell your troubles how big your Higher Power is. That should scare them away.

Chapter 4
MOTHRA MEETS GODZILLA

When written in Chinese, the word "crisis" is
composed of two characters: one represents danger
and the other represents opportunity.
—John F. Kennedy (1917–1963)

♥ *Affirmation:* All of my relationships are loving and harmonious.

I didn't sleep a bit the prior night, and now, on the day of surgery, I find out that rather than being one of the first operations of the day, mine will be one of the last. I'm hungry from fasting, dazed from lack of sleep, and not in a good mood. I want this over with because the waiting is killing me.

Nervous butterflies that began in my gut last night while at a restaurant have morphed into Mothra, the Japanese moth monster. I'm expecting Godzilla any moment, to complete my inner destruction. People, including Peter, try to ignore my stomach's relentless noises.

Just when I think I can't feel any worse, it occurs to me that this will be the first time I'll have had surgery without my mother to read to me when I awaken or to care for me when I get home. The unbearable thought that I took her care for granted seizes my concentration. I don't want to cry — not here, not now. I might not stop. Great! Godzilla in the form of Mommy memories has just reared its ugly head and is rampaging through my mind instead of my stomach. *PMA!* I silently scream, *Positive mental attitude, think happy thoughts. Oh, God, this sucks! Please stop!*

Doctors come into the room to share surgery updates with parents and loved ones. "They were just benign polyps in her nose; she'll be awake soon" "His surgery went well and everything was negative." "If you'll follow me you can see him in recovery."

Each time I hear a positive result I know, even though I try hard to control my thoughts and stay positive, that my results will not be good. *Third time is a charm, Kathy, and you will be Dr. Wagner's third surgery, blah, blah, blah.* Despite my mental efforts, a tiny voice screams, *"Prepare yourself! Incoming!"* A warning of impending war.

I distract myself with an article about an amazing woman who also lives on Cape Cod. She had a seven-centimeter malignant tumor removed from her pelvic area and told the doctors to administer chemotherapy in the incision during surgery. She had regular chemotherapy, too. After each treatment in Boston she returned to Cape Cod and sat on the sand dunes with her husband, even in the snow, and healed. Her story is such an inspiration. If she could do that, anyone can, right? *What am I thinking? I don't have cancer, do I? That's enough! Stop those negative thoughts! Stop thinking, period!*

When my name is finally called, I practically jump up and run for the processing area. I can't wait for Valium to stop my incessant thoughts and the anesthetic to bring sweet, dreamless sleep.

"Most lumps in women are benign," the anesthesiologist reassures. She peers over her black-rimmed glasses, gives me a quick checkup, and fills out paperwork on her clipboard. "You can wear those lovely socks until you go into surgery, then you'll have to wear the ones provided by the hospital. You'll be covered with a warm blanket, so you don't need to worry about being chilled." She is mistaking my shivers for cold, but my trembling is from fear and hunger — mostly fear. Godzilla is still on the loose.

So much for my cashmere socks. I'll hide them under the blanket. "May I please have some Valium now? I'm really anxious." I wring my hands for effect.

"Sure. We'll try to make you comfortable. Just lie back and relax," she replies with a smile. "More people from my team will come in to see you before surgery."

Seconds later, an Asian man in blue surgical scrubs enters the little cubicle and babbles something — then waits during a very pregnant pause.

Grabbing Peter's shirtsleeve, I whisper, "What did he say?"

"I think he said he's your nurse anesthetist or phlebotomist or something. I'm not sure," he whispers. "And I think he wants your socks."

Not my socks! They are safely hidden beneath the warming blanket, so how does he even know about them? Actually, I don't care. I want Valium, now. To expedite getting it, I decide to barter. With my nicest smile and sweetest voice, I jokingly tell him I will trade my socks for Valium and inquire if he is Japanese.

"No!" He barked. The big smile is gone. "Chinese!" He yanks my socks off with one swift motion and hands them like strangled chickens to Peter, who promptly stuffs them into his coat pocket. I'm flabbergasted and frightened, and my feet are cold.

I've just insulted a man holding a huge needle that will be going into my arm, possibly many times. I wonder what I was thinking, and decide to beg, barter having failed. I beg in earnest, he barks in response. This continues until Peter explains that the nurse anesthetist is explaining that he will give me the Valium intravenously. After three tries and a shot of Novocain to numb my hand, I finally get my Valium. *Oh, yes. I feel much, much, better.* As I'm wheeled off to surgery my husband kisses my hand and face and tells me he loves me.

"I'll be right here when you come out," he whispers, hunched over the gurney, following as far as the nurses will allow.

Well on my way to la-la land, I feel the best I have in weeks, no dreams, voices, or anxiety attacks. Mothra and Godzilla are dancing, and I can't feel my feet. I'll be asleep before I get to ask Dr. Wagner about the MRI. Guess I'll know soon enough.

As I drift off I wonder about grief, illness, and survival: *Statistics state that grief can cause illness. A broken heart can be deadly. Can a broken heart be seen on an MRI? How long does it take to mend a broken heart, Mom?*

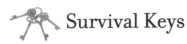 Survival Keys

✳ Laugh until it heals.

✳ Learn to dance in the rain. Life isn't about waiting
  for the endless storms to pass; it's about learning to
  dance in the rain.

✳ Face setbacks knowing you will move forward. It will
  often seem like you will take two steps forward only
  to take one step back.

Chapter 5

VALIDATION

*Our worst nightmares are blessings in disguise. They are a
microcosm of our waking world and inner guidance. Find the
pearl of wisdom, change the ending and change your life for the
better forever. Then wear your pearls with pride.*
— Kathleen O'Keefe-Kanavos

♥ *Affirmation:* When I make a decision, I choose to believe that the
universe will conspire to make it happen.

"Okay, let's close her up." Dr. Wagner's voice echoes down a dark tunnel of black, drug-induced sleep, where I've been floating in suspended animation. I claw my way toward consciousness, light, and, sound.

"What is it?" I ask, dragging myself up over a ledge of anesthesia. Light blinds me as I turn to face him. The blue eyes above his mask fly open and the medical personnel stare in disbelief.

"Did she just speak?" a voice asks from above my head. I gaze up at someone peering down at me. Thankfully, he is blocking the overhead light.

"It's, it's just what we thought, Kathy — a fibrosis tumor," Dr. Wagner stammers, still frozen in shock, gloved hands held high, eyes wide as if having seen a ghost.

I groan from the most excruciating pain I've ever experienced, but manage to smile through gritted teeth and say, "Oh, good."

"Give her more, now!" are the last words I hear as I slide back into the dark hole of anesthesia and resume floating.

The first warning bell tolls in my brain when Dr. Wagner pulls the privacy curtain behind him in the little recovery cubicle. The second one gongs when he takes my hand. "Pathology didn't like what they saw when they cut the tumor open," he says. The shock momentarily replaces nausea with panic.

"Is it cancer?" I hold fast to the side of the gurney and brace myself for the answer I already suspect.

"Yes, I'm sorry. I'll get your husband and refer you to a specialist."

The specialist I requested in your office when you told me I was too young for cancer?

So my voices and dreams had been right, the doctors and tests wrong. With my surgeon's words, the first shot of my ensuing battle is fired, and not a warning shot, but a point-blank bullet to my breast. I glance down at my painful wound and weep.

Thus begins my descent down the dark rabbit hole of Cancerland. There is no returning to my previous life. Like Alice, I'm falling, falling with no bottom in sight and little hope of a soft landing. The dream of dolphins just the night before now makes sense. I understand the people who surrounded the aggressive man. Pathology didn't see him until those containing him were cut away. I think about my dream of the secretary with the list. Didn't she say that I had let this go on for too long and now it was in everything? *Oh, God! I think I'm in big trouble.* My dreams had tried to prepare me for what pathology had just validated. I have cancer!

The dreams that drove me crazy also drove me to action and, I hope, will save my life. That must be the silver lining, if there is a silver lining to being diagnosed with a life-threatening disease. I focus on that positive thought but cry louder.

Peter slips silently through the curtain into my cubicle and throws his arms around me. We cry without regard for anyone who may be unnerved by the sound of our sorrow. I know patients can hear through the thin curtain as we sob, but we're too devastated to care. The bullet cannot be called back. Unfortunately, my husband can't stay in the recovery room with me because my nausea has returned tenfold, as much from the anesthesia as the dire news with its accompanying terror. A nurse attaches a bag of anti-nausea medication to my IV and offers me a paper cup of ginger ale, the smell of which gives me the dry heaves. In my recovery chair, bags of many colors hang above my head like a Dr. Seuss Christmas tree. A woman smiles from the end of a row of chairs, but when I try to smile back, the corners of my mouth won't turn up. Just when I think I will dissolve into another puddle of tears, the woman beside me asks, "What perfume are you wearing, dear? You smell so good." At first shocked, I then laugh through my sobs and reply, "Surgical scrub soap." It did smell nice.

While in recovery, I speak to the voices in my head. *"You were right about removing that damn spot. I should have acted sooner. Thank you and please don't leave me now."*

"You're welcome. We won't."

I'm scared out of my mind and realize how much I need those voices. If I am to win this war, I need a viable weapon beyond the medical community, which has let me down. Had I not been a squeaky wheel, I'd be dying right now. Hell, I might be dying anyway. *Shhh!* My guides armed me with powerful feathers once. I hope they have more where those came from in case I need them in the future — if I still have a future.

With that thought, I finally stop crying and slip into an exhausted slumber.

When we get home I call Jeanne in Virginia Beach to arrange a psychic reading from Sama Ling, a "sleeping channel" with whom she has worked. Jeanne was one of the instructors at the Psychic Academy in Virginia Beach that Peter had attended ten years before. One of her protégés was Sama Ling, who, while in a meditative induced trance, gives medical readings. He has quite a following because of his accuracy.

Channeling is what happened to Whoopi Goldberg in the movie *Ghost*. Until now, I had not been interested in channeling. In fact, I never really wanted to do anything psychic, despite being a closet intuitive. Psychics were not sanctioned by the Church, so they were not sanctioned by Mom. Therefore I hid my intuitive side. But once married to Peter, I began to question the reservations Mom had about psychics. At a workshop in Tampa I met Sama Ling. We did remote viewings. One person held a picture out of sight of a partner, who had to describe it. A stranger to me held a picture of a rose, which I described down to the dew on the petals and its likeness to the style of Monet. Having enjoyed the class, I finally embraced my inner psychic.

Fortunately, Sama Ling remembered me now and gave a reading that said I should de-compartmentalize my life and that the doctors would cure me, but it would be up to me to stay healthy. Okay, the curing part sounds good, but what is de-compartmentalizing and how is it done?

The reading over, I phone Jeanne and my emotional floodgates open. Everything I had been feeling, *and hearing*, pours out. As always, she listens patiently until I run out of information and breath, and then offers to continue helping with my dream interpretations during treatment. Jeanne also suggests I keep a journal next to my bed so I can immediately write down my dreams in the morning and not forget them. (As if I could, even if I tried.) Jeanne cautions that my dreams might become more frightening, but that their information could be a blessing in disguise. She also encourages me to look up her spiritually adopted daughter, Cindy, a doctor at the Children's Hospital in Boston and a Reiki master. Reiki, Jeanne explains, is a form of healing that uses spiritual energy. Although this is the first I've heard of it, I believe spiritual healing can really work. I know that dreams do.

I remember how much I enjoyed Peter's dream-therapy classes in Virginia Beach. I believe dreams are the windows to our inner selves and that through them we can communicate with ourselves and loved ones. It is the way your inner ET (Eternal Teacher) can phone home to the other side for help. This seems true with the dreams I'd had lately. My psychic school lessons are now being put to the test, as am I. I'll need everything in my survival arsenal, conventional and unconventional, to win this war. Who would have thought that lessons learned decades ago in a school I never intended to attend would now help me save my life?

Shortly after we married, I accompanied Peter to a psychic academy in Virginia Beach so he could study channeling and giving medical readings, similar to Sama Ling's, while I visited former army-brat friends. I had no interest in the academy. Channeling seemed like controlled schizophrenia to me. Neither the instructors nor my husband had any idea that I was intuitive. I had always described myself as a "sensitive-sensitive."

"What the hell is a sensitive-sensitive?" Peter had asked.

"I'm very sensitive to everything and everyone. That's why I smell things you can't smell and hear sounds you can't hear." He'd seen my nose and ears in action many times as I described the layers of smells from people encircling him.

Yet while at this academy in Virginia Beach, I found it refreshing to be in a roomful of people and be able to say, "Hi. My name is Kathy, and I'm a Sensitive," and hear the response: "Hi, Kathy, so are we," and know that these voices were not in my head.

I had avoided the word "psychic." Discussing such a thing was not encouraged in my family, even though my grandparents were well-known spiritualists. That was a family secret, something one kept in the closet with the other family skeletons — such as murder.

It was in Virginia Beach that Peter found out how sensitive I really am. "We're a match made in heaven," he later said. Any other man would have run for the hills.

I remember the very evening this realization took place. It had begun with an introduction to the instructors and ended with a psychic class meeting so everyone could meet Peter, the new student. I had been invited to attend by instructors Jeanne and Jason.

"We would have enrolled you in the class with Peter but we only take psychic students," Jeanne says with an apologetic smile, and hands us the keys to our rental condo. Christopher, her silver Persian cat, jumps into my lap, looking into my face with his golden eyes. "He likes you," Jeanne says.

"He says he doesn't feel well," I answer.

"Oh, he suffers from allergies," Jason replies, shooting a quick glance at Jeanne.

"I completely understand," I respond to Jeanne's previous comment about enrollees, my intuitions hidden behind a thick wall. "I'll be busy with friends."

Reading the list of things Peter is required to do daily to encourage his abilities, I'm downright relieved to be excluded. I know psychics who would do all Peter's fasting, soaking, and much more if they thought it would make them non-psychic, but it wouldn't change a thing. They'd still be psychics, just psychics in denial. I know because that described Mom and me, but if you are born with perceptive insight, and I believe we all are (we learn not to be sensitive), training can increase intuition. The academy was a wonderful place to study phenomena like dream therapy, synchronicities, and spiritual guides. I believe everyone has and should be in touch with her or his spirit guides. We're their job. And they take their job seriously.

One evening, the class sits around an empty chair. *This is pretty intimidating,* I think. *I wonder who sits there?* That was where they put Peter. Then they proceed to close their eyes and put their palms out to "feel" him. Finally, they give their impressive impressions. Peter is unanimously accepted into the class.

"Would Kathy be willing to sit in the seat and let us feel her? She looks like our daughter-in-law," a friendly couple asks. Jeanne looks at me.

As I sit in the hot seat, I "open myself" and proceed to heat up the room to a state of discomfort. Everyone asks me to shut down while they peel off clothing and open doors. "Sorry. I opened so you could read me." I, too, am accepted and attend dream classes, but as a dreamer who forgets details, I get three tips from Jeanne to remember my dreams:

Keep a notebook beside the bed.

In the morning write down something, even if it's only a feeling — happy, sad, frightened — and any color associated with the dream.

Then give the dream a title.

"This helps open the doors to your dream memory," Jeanne explains.

After Peter's initiation, we return to our tiny condo with twin beds in separate rooms. My bedroom also has a friendly one-legged cricket

I name Jiminy. The previous renter had thrown a shoe and knocked off one of his legs, making for a quiet bug. Jiminy would crawl from his hiding place and eat the crumbs I offered while I told him about my dream classes. "Who are you talking to?" Peter called from the other bedroom.

"Just my cricket." I could imagine Peter's look of angst.

It was a cozy condo but a difficult place to sleep. As I drift off, Indian chants and bells begin around my bed. After the fourth chant and bell session, I sit up and say, "Thank you for the lovely charms, but please stop so I can dream for my journal."

"Who are you talking to, now?" Peter groans from the other bedroom.

"Just the Indians."

"Bunny, go back to sleep."

Dreams are not the only things that hold pearls of wisdom. Jeanne encourages students to discover answers that worked for them in their life and level of learning. She says, "We are always exactly where we must be in life. We cannot, at this time or moment, be anywhere else.

More than a decade later, I'm using that Psychic Academy education to survive crisis. How many other of those students are using dream "baby steps" to communicate with their guides during crisis? Were we at the academy back then because that was exactly where we needed to be for our future? And is this all synchronicity, divination, divine intervention, or just plain luck? Only time will tell.

Survival Keys

* Use conventional methods and intuitive guidance.
  Both can be lifesaving. Given a choice, take both.
  Why limit yourself?

* Believe but validate. Cross checking for confirmation
  gives a level of knowledge greater than the sum of the
  individual parts.

* Remember: You are spirit inhabiting a body to have a
  human experience. Surviving crisis is part of life on
  earth.

* Know we all have Spirit Guides/Guardian Angels. We
  are their job; they take their job seriously, and speak
  to us through dreams, meditations, and prayer.

* Embrace conventional and spiritual guidance easily
  by loving both.

Chapter 6

IN CRISIS, DEEP BREATHS

It's the Cheshire Cat: now I shall have someone to talk to.
"How are you getting on?" said the Cat as soon as there
was mouth enough to speak with.
— Alice in Wonderland

♥ *Affirmation:* I will promote what I love
rather than bash what I dislike.

Breathe! I tell myself as the room spins and my ears ring. Since my operation, I unconsciously hold my breath. I don't even realize it until I become dizzy. Only then, on the verge of fainting, is there temporary relief from my horrific reality. *I might die! My mother died of cancer! Breathe!* With another gulp of air, I distract myself from my fear and clean an already spotless kitchen counter for the fourth or fifth time. I can't remember because I can't concentrate long enough to count. *"Breathe, deep breaths, Kathy, deep breaths,"* the voice yelled as I tried to overcome another anxiety attack. No matter how much air I breathe, it doesn't seem to be enough, and I claw at my throat.

I know anxiety attacks. I've had them while scuba diving at ninety feet in the open ocean with sharks. I mastered panic then. I can do it now, while facing a different type of deadly predator. This is yet another page from my Life Lesson's Book applied to my current predicament. *How to Survive Panic Attacks: From Deadly Sharks to Deadlier Cancer.*

Dr. Wagner phones to reassure us that the preliminary pathology report looks positive. The tumor appears to be less than two centimeters, which is in the beginning of stage one. "Early stage cancer is very treatable," he reassures us. "I don't expect anything to be in the lymph nodes." My next procedure is scheduled with a surgical oncologist (the specialist I requested at my first surgery) to check for clean margins and determine if all the cancer was removed. *BREATHE!*

I'm having trouble hearing my doctor's voice on the phone. (Is this hysterical deafness, the sibling of hysterical blindness?) What's worse than being diagnosed with a life-threatening illness? Waiting for the final pathology report to find out just how sick you really are. *Breathe, Kathy. Breathe!*

Why me? The question won't be ignored so I meditate and get an interesting answer.

"Why not! You are part of Team Earth where the ultimate goal is to experience life until you die. This is part of your destiny and earthbound experience." What's that saying—"He who dies with the most toys wins"? I never fully understood that before, but unfortunately, it's starting to make perfect sense. The rules of the game sound so simple, but I don't want to play anymore. Rather than fight this disease, I want to run away and hide, take my bat and ball and go home. Actually, I could jump into my car and bolt, but how would that help? It's not like running away from an abusive relationship or an unbearable job. The problem is a physical part of me. No matter where I go, there I'll be…with "it." There's only one place I can go where it cannot follow, because I'll leave my body and *crisis* behind. I could hang myself. There's that dark thought again.

"Get hold of yourself, Kathy. Do you really want to leave? You can. But what a waste, because I don't think your guides would fight like this for you if they didn't think you could win. It may be very hard, but so is life. And remember: difficulty, pain, or bad luck is relative and a matter of perception. So what's it gonna be? Fight or flight? Live or die? We all have to be together in this decision, because if we don't hang together, we'll hang together," my inner selves say. The silence is tangible as they wait for my answer.

Hanging may be too scary. What if I don't do it right? There are enough pills in the medicine cabinet to kill an elephant; many of them left over from Mom's fight with cancer. I'm still not ready to part with anything I have left of her. Medicine bottles with her name on them reassure me life with her was not a dream. I even keep a plastic Ziploc bag of her favorite clothes in my closet. When I miss her so much that I can't function, I open the bag and breathe in her smells — a "hit of Mama." It would be so easy to take all those pills with some nice vodka, then lie on the bed, pull a plastic bag over my head, go to sleep, and wake up with someone who experienced what I'm going through and will understand — Mom.

One of my inner selves is a fighting Irish (who loves vodka martinis), and she never gives up. She will beat a dead horse for a very long time and immediately ruins my plastic-bag-over-the-head plan by pointing out an important fact I'd failed to consider: *"If you kill yourself, Mom will be waiting for us and kick our butts around Heaven like a football. She fought to the end!"*

She's right. Okay. *Plan A: We'll stay and fight with all our inner and outer resources! I refuse to allow this crisis to be my cruel, manipulating Svengali. We'll file the flight plan of pills, booze, and bags under plan Y or Z. I think we just took a big step. We're united and have a game plan:* FIGHT *and* LIVE!

All this mental babble is exhausting, so I crawl off to take a nap. I grimace from pain and try to find a comfortable spot. I'm still so sore from surgery. Baby Cakes climbs up behind me, gently rests his head on mine, wraps his paws around my neck, and purrs away. As I meditate on returning my body to perfection, I hear Baby Cakes echo that thought in my ear, "Puurfect, puurfect." He has done this quite often lately, and when he does, I become so relaxed I forget having fallen asleep or dreaming, such a treat. But tonight I have a lucid dream. My spirit guides arm me with mystical weapons for my upcoming battle. I name it My Color and Number.

In this dream there are two locks on my hotel room door but I want more. I phone a maintenance man to install a third. In the lobby, two girlfriends hug and ask me to join them in the lounge to dance. First I must get my two cats from my husband's room, because he doesn't have good locks on his door. Then I run down a hallway full of people toward my room.

Later, I join my friends, but sit alone at a round table while they writhe on their backs on the floor to music. Their mini-dresses ride up, and their undergarments are visible while they get their shoes cleaned by an electric shoe machine. I wonder if this is acceptable behavior, when a voice beside me says, "If the underclothes are attractive why not show them?" I agree and see a friendly Gypsy seated at my table. She holds up a large, glittery yellow-gold piece of Egyptian papyrus with writing that changes hue as the paper moves. She reads aloud from it: "Your number is two and your color is orange."

I ask why there are different hues on the paper. "It is so everyone can see," she replies. Since the Gypsy seems to have all the answers, I ask her about my mother, but she rolls her eyes at me and doesn't answer, so I leave.

Interpretation: This mystical dream shows resolve to take control of a health situation, but most important it demonstrates that I am not alone and have the support of spirit guides who empower me with spiritual gifts. I wouldn't be surprised if I have just met some of the voices in my head that I've encountered during my waking hours and daydreams. The message is clear: "Don't worry, be happy," and "This gift's for you."

Taking Jeanne's earlier suggestion, I phone Cindy, the Boston pediatrician. She invites us to her Chinese New Year party. I love parties. I just hope my Chinese anesthetist isn't there. Wouldn't that be a kick?

It's the year of the rabbit, which has always been associated with strong lunar symbolism and intuition. This probably arose from the rabbit's habit of suddenly bounding up from its hiding place, as intuitive messages often do. In mythology the rabbit appears as a supernatural figure giving advice for life changes. Sounds like my kind of year, with Mom's full moon as a special symbol of love for me, and my white rabbit intuition in full swing.

I "get Reikied" for the first time at Cindy's party, and it feels great. I can feel the warm energy emanating from her hands. As I sit in a chair, she passes her hands over my chakras and spends extra time on my right breast. The area gets very warm, so I know something is happening. She calls this a "Reiki boost," a technique used when a Reiki table is not available. She explains that Reiki uses the universal healing energy or God energy. It is never depleted and keeps the healer from getting burned out. Once home, I look up information about Reiki on the Internet. It is a healing modality discovered in Sanskrit writings by a Japanese teacher, Mikao Usui, while on a mission to discover the process Jesus Christ and other great healers used to heal.

The biggest challenges that need to be overcome at this point in my healing process are fear of the unknown and feeling out of control. Reiki offers two keys to survival by giving you self-healing tools and creating a sense of self-control over your healing process. The difference between Reiki and other healing modalities is the attunement process, which creates a pathway for energy flow and can also be used for self-healing.

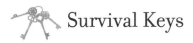 ## Survival Keys

* Explore modalities. Don't be afraid to research and try healing techniques such as Reiki, which has a long tradition.

* Remember that we create our hell or heaven.

Chapter 7

DANCING IN THE EYE
OF THE STORM

I can't go back to yesterday—
because I was a different person then.
— Alice in Wonderland

♥ *Affirmation:* I believe that God will not give me
anything I cannot handle.

The party is over. I'm sitting on the examining table in Dr. Kritchen's office, awaiting my official, and hopefully final, pathology report. I'm so anxious my feet won't be still. This is my new emotional roller-coaster ride. I thought my nerves were bad in the waiting room, but this is far worse. My heart is racing, and my blood pressure is 154 over 94. My normal pressure is 117 over 72. My ears pound as my right eye and leg twitch. This constant hurry-up-and-wait reminds me of life in the military. How did Mom handle this anxiety when she received her death sentence? Will I now receive mine? It's frightening to think Mom's past situation is now my present one. Am I just feeling sorry for myself and acting like a big baby? Well, I'm about to wet my pants, and I just used the bathroom seconds ago.

Dr. Wagner had referred us to Dr. Kritchen, Head of Surgical Oncology, who looks like Alice's Cheshire cat, with an ear-to-ear grin and a rotund body. I feel like a combination of the white rabbit and Alice: I'm late, I'm late! Hurry up and take this pill or eat that piece of kombucha mushroom, and let's see what happens. Maybe I'll get well,

38

or maybe I'll slowly disappear, a body part at a time, starting with my breasts. And while we wait to see what happens, let's continue the Mad Tea Party of examining tables. Everyone grab a gown and move down one room, and don't forget the dormouse — we'll need it for the hundreds of computer printouts they'll stuff into my file. This is my new reality: half fairytale, half reality crouched on examining tables, twitching like a rabbit and watching the clock in hopes that I'm not *too* late. But for what? Well now, that's the *real* question, isn't it? We'll soon find out.

Dr. Kritchen enters the room with his grin, waves my pathology report above his head, and does a soft-shoe as he spins around. This has to be good news. Maybe I don't need to have my breast removed. The bad news: I still need a second surgery to check for clear margins and lymph nodes. So, today's *final* pathology report has been moved down to my *next-to-final report* as the Mad Tea Party continues. The report also showed the tumor as 2.1 centimeters, the beginning of stage-2 cancer — not 1 centimeter or stage-1 cancer.

More coulda-woulda-shoulda sets in. I should have had an oncology surgeon perform, or be present at, my first surgery. Maybe then I wouldn't need this second surgery. Sitting on the table now, I remember asking Dr. Wagner, "Who is doing my surgery?" and again, his answer, "I am. An oncologist won't be necessary." I wonder if the anxiety I felt at the time was my spiritual guides/gut instincts screaming at me. Why did I not listen again? Would I ever learn to listen, or must I always take classes at the University of Hard Knocks. Well, when I finish this course in Cancer 101, I will graduate with a doctorate in Voices and Crisis Management. My thesis will be *Voices: To Listen or Not to Listen, That is the Question.*

Yes, a biopsy while the lump was still pea-sized would have helped to determine whether:

I needed an oncology surgeon or surgery at all.

The lump was benign or malignant.

Had I known this then, I'd have run to the nearest oncologist, with or without an appointment, as soon I felt my hard spot, before it had time to grow into the problem it is today. I've learned the hard way to be my own squeaky-wheel-pain-in-the-ass self-advocate. Needle biopsies, I've heard from other friends, are relatively painless. Sitting on this examining table four months after I first found my lump is extremely painful. And this second surgery won't be painless either. Live and learn.

"You are where you are in life because that is exactly where you need to be at this moment." Jeanne's words from Virginia Beach ring in my ears. Maybe I should stop beating myself up for my past errors and learn from them so I can move forward. Forgiveness is freedom. Holding grudges or negativity allows someone despicable to live rent-free in your mind. Forgiveness evicts them with love.

Voices can be tricky. I remember Buffy, a special-needs student, turning to me in reading class and calmly saying, "My people in my head told me to kill you."

"Well, you tell those people in your head your teacher says no, and that they are to get out of your head right now and never, ever come back because that is unacceptable behavior."

"Okay," she answered, and never mentioned them again.

So, when do you listen to "the voices" and when do you tell them to shut up? When they tell you to do something harmful, tell them to take a hike. But, let's get back to "being where you are right now because that is where you should be in order to grow." Here are some invaluable lessons I learned in my Class from Hell at the University of Hard Knocks, AKA UHK.

Life Lesson #1: Go to the professionals who handle specific problems. Don't play the wait-and-see game. It can have deadly consequences, and you'll seldom win.

Life Lesson #2: Go somewhere reputable for mammograms, because they're only as good as the people who take and read them, so both of these medical personnel need to be well trained.

"How did the multiple mammograms and doctors miss a stage-2 tumor in the first place?" I asked Dr. Kritchen. He put the mammogram film up on a backlit wall and showed exactly how "it didn't show up." The mammogram was so dark it looked like a waxing gibbous moon and dark shadows, a result of young, dense breasts. I wondered if I found the shadows indistinguishable because I'm not trained in reading mammograms, but I realized by the strained look on Dr. Kritchen's face that he can't read them either.

Life Lesson #3: Yell and scream if lessons 1 and 2 don't put your gut instincts at ease, even though the test results are within the normal range, because,

Life Lesson #4: There are no norms. There is only you. Be your own advocate. When voices/intuition communicates with you, listen! They are seldom there for chitchat. I ignored my inner voices when they spoke concerning my mother's impending death. The signs were all there during the hour of souls. It may be time to open that locked door deep in the bowels of my mind and revisit that awful night full of the signs and symbols — the night my mother died.

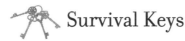 ## Survival Keys

* ✳ Seek a second opinion or self-advocate when your gut instincts are at odds with conventional information, doctors, authorities, or therapists.

* ✳ Know that second opinions can be lifesavers.

* ✳ Learn that you are responsible for yourself. It's okay to be difficult when necessary for survival.

* ✳ Don't allow yourself to be dismissed.

* ✳ Be a squeaky wheel until you are heard.

Chapter 8

HOUR OF SOULS

There are none so blind as those who will not see.
—Jeremiah 5:12, the Holy Bible, King James Version

♥ *Affirmation:* Grief is love. I choose love, joy and freedom. Open my heart and allow wonderful things to flow into my life.

The moon was full the night my mother died. The colon cancer won, as she silently surrendered her body during the hour of souls, that special time between 2:00 and 4:00 a.m., different from the witching hour of midnight. Mom had always described it as the time when souls in hospitals often chose to free themselves of their bodies. As a nurse and a psychic-in-denial because of her Catholic convent upbringing, Mom had seen enough people die to know it was a special time for death. Did she choose to die during this hour, or did it just happen? Do we have control over our time of death, or are we suddenly in a dream from which we cannot awaken, unaware of our passing? Most important, are we alone, confused, and frightened?

After the dreadful call, I sat outside on my deck chair in the dark. Numb with grief, hugging my knees to my chest and rocking for comfort while mulling over these questions until they transformed into a physical knot in the pit of my stomach. Receiving no answers, I turned those thoughts inward to my weeklong emotional blindness. All the signs of impending death had stared me in the face, yet I ignored Death waving at me in the distance. Would things have happened differently tonight if I had understood those unearthly signals as messages from the other side? Mom saw them, as did her nurse.

42

Where are you Mom, really, where are you right now? My mind screams as much to myself as to her. I didn't want to think *she's in a better place in heaven, with God and Jesus, blah, blah, and blah*.... Emotions reached a crescendo of confusion compounded by grief and immense guilt: *What kind of daughter would pray for her mother's death? Did I do this to Mom with prayers that begged God to either heal or steal her? Was Mom's death the power of prayer, the circle of life, or both?*

Would a Higher Power actually listen to someone as insignificant as me with all that is happening in this world? *You are using this God thought as a distraction from the real question at hand. Answer the question! What kind of daughter would pray for her mother's death?* I hug my legs even tighter and cry into my knees. A voice whispers, "*A daughter whose love has no limits or boundaries.*" I sit motionless, then rotate in the chair, eyes and ears straining to locate the elusive voice. Is someone else here? I need to speak to that voice because right now the "afterlife" seems like some pathetic fairytale. I feel Mom's soul is at stake. "Mom! Where are you?" I whisper, then strain again to hear the voice in the breeze.

Uprooted frequently, we spent so much time together while my military father traveled to places too far or dangerous for us to follow. We were often our only source of comfort and friendship... strangers in strange lands. Surely Mom would answer me now if she could. Was she now a stranger in another strange land, alone, confused, and looking for me as I called out for her? Did she know she was dead yet? How far away could she possibly be with only an hour separating her from life? Then, the ultimate question of life and death pushed its ugly head to the surface of my mind from the deepest, darkest depths of my despair. *If I died right now, could I catch up to her? Could I find my mom? Could we offer each other comfort?*

Stop that thought right now! I scolded myself. *What are you thinking? Get a grip!*

I taught psychology at the University of South Florida, and I knew that that particular question was always dangerous, especially when one is consumed by grief. Such thoughts could get you locked away on suicide watch. But I wasn't being suicidal — just honest in my curiosity about this afterlife concept. Would the elusive voice chide me for my dangerous curiosity or agree with me. All I hear are palm fronds rustling in the tropical breeze. Maybe the answer is too dangerous for a mere mortal to understand. After all, it really is a lovely night to die.

I wipe the stream of tears from my face with the sleeve of my silk nightshirt and notice the reflection of the full moon shimmering in our swimming pool, so close yet so far. Could this moon connect Mom to me now? Was there no way to ever again pick up a telephone and say, "Hey, Mom, want to go get lunch and chat?" The reality of this "past life" in my present state makes me sick to my stomach. I sit perfectly still and will the waves of nausea to pass — afraid to even move my eyes from the glow of the silvery moon.

I should have been there holding her hand when she died. The thought of her dying alone is more unbearable than the thought of her dying at all. She would never have left me alone.

Was my absence fueled by a fear of death, or was it an unspoken mutual agreement decided before our births and only now remembered and played out so she could leave this earth and I could let her go? Was the thought of losing my mother, my best friend and mentor, a person I had loved all my life, too devastating to handle? Would watching her die emotionally destroy me for life, or would the profound grief she would have seen on my face at the moment of her death hold her here on the earth plane past her time and prolong her suffering?

The first sign tonight that all was not well was when Mom told me there was a man in the hospital room, whom no one else could see, watching her. She refused to let the nurses undress her in front of him and clutched the sheets tightly around her frail body while staring at a corner by the window at the foot of her bed. The nurses dismissed her behavior as a reaction to the meds in her IV drip. "It's just a drug-induced hallucination," they whispered. "We see it all the time."

"Mom, do you know the man? Have you seen him before? Does he talk to you?"

"No," she answered, clear as a bell to all three questions. "He just stands there and watches me. He's there right now," she said, pointing with her nose because both weak, bruised arms were taped with multiple IVs, lifelines to a dying cause. Looking at the dark window, I was startled by an unrecognizable reflection — mine. It was weary, with deep circles etched beneath sunken eyes. My ever-present dark sunglasses were pushed back on my head. I never knew when I might need to flip them down to hide tears. No one else was at the foot of Mom's bed.

Despite my psychic gifts, I was too emotionally numb to feel this invisible person. All my emotional and intuitive buttons were turned down to deal rationally with the present crisis. However, the notion of this unseen man conjured up new questions. *"Is Mr. Invisible here to protect Mom, take her from me, or catch a ride with her if she goes to the other side?* Questions instantly dismissed as too deep for my emotionally saturated mind to ponder. I'll save them for another time, when I can handle the answers.

Mom described her invisible visitor as young, of medium height, with straight, short brown hair and brown eyes. This description didn't sound like a hallucination. Mom was more lucid tonight than she had been in days. The morphine drip only numbed her body.

Whenever the doctor came into Mom's room and announced with a smile, "We'll clear up Mom's pneumonia, and she'll be back home to resume chemotherapy in a week," I'd flip down my dark sunglasses, slink off to the nearest bathroom, sit on a toilet seat, and cry as silently as possible. I had suspected when I checked Mom into the hospital five days earlier that she would not check out in the conventional way. No loving family members would wheel her out to a car and finally to a comfy bed at home. I didn't want to think about how and to where she would finally be wheeled by strangers just doing their jobs. It wouldn't be warm and comfy.

Deep inside, I always suspected the doctor's medically predicted happy ending was not to be our reality. The invisible man in the room tonight confirmed this. But rather than reading signs, I ignored them with blind denial, even when Mom tried to tell me that her colon cancer was the only cancer that had ever been in our family. That conversation had taken place the day before this during another unusually lucid moment.

"I don't know how much more time I have," she said, gently holding my hand. Her cold gurney was pushed against the corridor wall as she waited for an ultrasound to confirm what she already knew, but I refused to accept — the degree to which the cancer had metastasized.

During her procedure, Mom looked intently into my eyes for my reaction. I flipped down my sunglasses. I didn't want to increase her pain by having to watch me suffer. The test confirmed that her sands of time were down to a few stubborn grains clinging to the side of her hourglass.

That evening, while I helped the aide change Mom's soiled gown and sheets for the fifth time, the nurse asked me if I planned to stay the night.

"Stay the night?" I repeated. She knew I lived only minutes away. She smiled that smile that comes from years of experience with death, then continued her rounds and left me to ponder her question. I wanted to believe that I would see Mom again the next morning to groom her hair and tuck a pillow behind her sore back, so, as I applied a damp cloth to her closed eyes, and the overhead fluorescent lights created a halo around her, I leaned over and kissed her goodnight. Despite the oxygen tube, her breathing was so labored that she slept in an upright Buddha position and appeared to be deep in meditation. Looking back, I wonder if it might have been deeper than meditation. Perhaps another sign I had missed.

Now, in the glow of the full moon, I realize the nurse's question was sign number two. The nurse and Mom knew what I refused to see: Death had been coming closer.

It was 11:00 p.m. when I returned home emotionally and physically exhausted. My husband was in Tampa working on an important business deal, so I snuggled peacefully in bed with Baby Cakes and sought comfort in his purr while we watched Arnold Schwarzenegger blast jungle trees to pieces with an M134 Minigun in *Predator*. Suddenly, three huge dark shadows entered the bedroom through the pool area's locked sliding-glass door, slid across the ceiling, and flew down the hallway toward the room my mother had occupied for the past six weeks. The dark blobs appeared to be searching for something.

"What the hell was that?" I yelled and ducked beneath the covers. I heard Baby Cakes jump off the bed and slide across the marble floor as he ran for my closet. *Nothing just flew around the room; there were no shadows on the ceiling*, I repeated as I peered from the safety of the sheets. What I should have done was jump out of bed and speed back to the hospital, but I was still immersed in denial and refusing to read the signs.

Peter arrived home after midnight. "You saw what? Where? You're overtired, Bunny," he said. "Let me hold you until you fall asleep." That had been his reaction to my flying blobs. But when he thought I wasn't looking, he peered down the hallway.

The shrill telephone woke us at 3:30 a.m., and a female voice gently announced that my mother had lost her fight. Now all the signs fit together like large pieces of a kindergarten jigsaw puzzle. They all made perfect sense: Mom's invisible man, the nurse asking me if I planned to stay the night, Mom's Buddha position, and the shadows on the ceiling. The signs were there, but I wasn't prepared to look at Death, even though Death had tried to make eye contact. However, Death is impossible to ignore when it slaps you in the face.

Now, drunk with grief and fatigue, I stagger back into bed and pull the covers protectively around my fetal position. I'm surprised, not by a voice but by what feels like invisible arms around me. Someone has snuggled against my back, "spooning" the way I, as a frightened child in Berlin, Germany, used to spoon against Mom, seeking protection from the nightly terror of marching ghost-soldiers in our haunted hallway. Cigarette smoke had filled the corridor during the witching hour and hour of souls of my childhood. Perfume fills it now.

It is the smell of Mom's perfume as she snuggles against me to offer comfort. She's still in my life, but on that other plane. I encircle my own body with my arms and hope that Mom can feel me hug her while she embraces me. She has just answered all my tortured questions with a simple act of love from the other side. Our souls will connect us forever across time, space, and realms. I don't need the phone or moon to unite us. If I listen, I will hear her. There are some things we can take with us; love is one of them.

Should I look for the signs I so carefully ignored during Mom's last days? Will my questions about the shadows on my bedroom ceiling be answered when they come to search for me?

The full moon became my shield against uncertainty, a personal symbol for survival and a sign of Mom's love. Anytime I gaze at it in the darkness of life, I whisper, "Look, Mom, there's our moon" and know in my heart that she hears me and smiles.

Baby boomers have become the generation of orphans. The three keys to surviving the loss of a loved one, especially a parent, are about understanding and embracing your emotions.

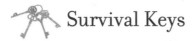 ## Survival Keys

* Realize it is natural for parents to die before their children. The mind may grasp what the heart cannot—the concept that parents die so children can "come into their own."

* Know that the death of a parent is an emotionally painful rite of passage.

* Grief is love. We do not grieve the loss of something we do not love. Love is an emotion that we can take with us to the other side and that unlocks many doors beyond time and space.

Chapter 9

TUMOR KILL AND TREATMENT TYPING

'But I don't want to go among mad people.' Alice remarked.
'Oh, you can't help that,' said the Cat. 'We're all mad here.'
— Alice in Wonderland

♥ *Affirmation:* I trust in the process of life.

On our way home from the appointment with Dr. Kritchen, we call
Peter's cousins in California with the news. They immediately share
the name and phone number of Dr. Robert A. Nagourney, the medical director of the Memorial Medical Cancer Center in Long Beach,
who does tumor kill and treatment typing. The tests, known as chemo
sensitivity and resistance assays, or CSRAs, test different chemotherapy drugs and combinations directly against a sample of the tumor to
identify which will be most effective in killing the tumor cells. They
also fax me a newspaper article explaining Dr. Nagourney's work. I
called Dr. Nagourney.

According to the doctor, chemo drugs in most hospitals are prescribed based on their overall performance in past trials, but even the
best drugs may fail to help 30 to 60 percent of patients. The article went
on to say that it is impossible to predict the outcome of a particular
cancer treatment for any individual because every cancer is different.
Dr. Nagourney said, "The average treatment for the average patient
can't possibly work all the time, because there are no average patients."

My thought exactly. He just confirmed lesson #4: There is no norm, only individuals.

There are two types of CSRAs: one that determines whether a drug stops a cancer's growth, and one that determines whether a drug kills the cancer outright. *That's the one I want!* Dr. Nagourney describes the case of a Cincinnati pathologist diagnosed with aggressive ovarian cancer. The standard treatment of Carboplatin and Taxol failed to stop it. She was dying, but sent samples of her tumor to Nagourney, who used the cell-death method and suggested the drugs Cisplatin and Gemzar. Three weeks later her cancer had disappeared.

Dr. Nagourney sent a kit to be refrigerated until the day of surgery, when a piece of tumor is placed into the kit and immediately sent back by express the next day. It took some convincing to get my Boston doctors to agree to use the kit, but to their credit, they did so when they found a cancerous lymph node. Peter posted it before I awoke from surgery. Within two weeks Dr. Nagourney would fax the results to my Boston oncologist, specifying which chemotherapy would work best for me. We asked Dr. Nagourney's office to please put a rush on it because, in the back of my mind, I still saw that hypodermic syringe filled with blood — the stick in the wasp's nest.

I'm having so many dreams now that I need a separate notebook for them. The thin veil between the realms of the living and the dead has definitely been pushed aside, because they appear to be more than normal nightly dreams. This night is no different.

I named this dream "The Room Between Realms."

Two guides step through a pop-up, flank me on either side, and lead me through a door into a white room that is devoid of furniture. The floor and ceiling meld together. They guide me through a roomful of people who stand in small groups and converse, but I cannot hear them. Spirit guides in front of and behind me lead other people who have also been brought to this place. They watch us pass by. Off to one side I see my mother talking to a group of women. I recognize one as the person who had appeared to me in my bedroom twenty years prior. I had had an adverse reaction to pain pills after my wisdom teeth were removed. The woman appears beside my bed along with two men who were out of sight, but whose laughter disturbed my sleep. She calls one Frank.

"Is she going to be okay?" Frank asks from the hallway.

"Yes, but she's in a lot of pain. It's good that she vomited those pills," the woman beside my bed answers as she leans over and peers down at me.

The next day I described to my mother the woman with blond, pageboy-style hair, wearing open-toed platform shoes and a puff-sleeved pleated dress with matching thin belt. She said, "That's your Aunt Evelyn and her husband Frank who always laughed. I think the man with Frank was his brother because they were inseparable." She should know. He was Mom's first husband. The sisters had married brothers to escape the convent.

Aunt Evelyn died of hypertension at age twenty-nine, fifteen years before I was born. The men were also dead. She checked on me two more times that night, twenty years ago, and now I was seeing her again, talking with Mom in my dream.

As my guides lead me past my mother, she turns from the group, waves, smiles, and slowly mouths the words "I love you." She does this twice.

"I can't hear her," I tell my guides. "I've heard her speak to me in my dreams before, so why can't I hear her now?" I look over my shoulder at Mom and try get out of the line, but the guides neither let me go nor stop.

"That is part of the process," one guide replies, and pulls me back through the pop-up into my original dream. Then both the door and the guides disappear.

Interpretation: This is a spirit-guided visit and a gift. I am taken through a room between time, space, dimensions, and realms to see my mother, about whom I had been worried since the day of her death and my diagnosis. My questions are finally answered: "Are you lonely, Mom? Are you happy and adjusting without us? Will we ever see each other again? Where are you right now?" Many of the same questions I had asked the night of her death. The guides show me that Mom is fine and is reunited with her sister and other loved ones. Now I can fully concentrate on myself and no longer worry about her. And the dream proves that love transcends time and space; you can take it with you.

It's so early this frigid Monday, and I'm not a morning person. The weather in Boston at the end of January is often stormy. I should be in Rancho Mirage, California, playing tennis in the warm sunshine and having lunch with friends, but instead I'm here at the hospital preparing for a second surgery. And once again I've insulted my Chinese nurse anesthetist by asking him if he is Japanese. Don't I ever learn? To make matters worse, I can't understand a word he's saying while he points that big needle at me. This is like bad déjà vu. I look closely to see if he is the same person I insulted at my first surgery. I don't think he is, but I'm not sure. Thank goodness Peter can interpret for me. "Tell him I want my Valium," I say as I tug on Peter's sleeve.

"Stop asking these people if they're Japanese! They're all Chinese, and you're insulting them," Peter whispered loudly out of the side of his mouth.

There is a reason I have such a fear of needles. As a child in Germany, I had had to get yearly shots in both of my little arms. These inoculations were required of all military dependents. "Please, please don't hurt me, Mr. Doctor," I would beg the corpsman as big tears streamed down my face and dripped off my quivering lower lip. I actually got a couple of those big strapping soldiers to cry with me, but they always gave me the injections. A grown man and a puny girl crying together was a scene that often drew spectators.

Peter's translation jolted me back into the moment. "The anesthetist is giving you a choice between general anesthesia and a spinal block."

A spinal block after I insulted him? I'd be wide-awake while the doctor cuts me. Is he crazy?! "First I want my Valium, then I want to be put out completely, and the sooner the better," I answer. My surgery will not be day surgery this time, because my sentinel lymph nodes must be tested with a blue dye. I'm not sure how that works, but it sure sounds strange. Anyway, the sooner I go to sleep the sooner the night in the hospital will pass and I can go home.

Back at home after my very first night in a hospital, it now seems unreal. I hope it will be my last. First, I was sicker than a dog from the anesthesia. Next, the night nurse gave me the wrong call button to summon her during the night. It was the TV control, so every time I used it to get help removing the inflatable boots that kept me from developing blood clots, so that I could go to the bathroom, I turned on the TV. Finally, at 1:00 a.m., on the verge of wetting the bed after my third attempt to contact the nurse by verbally calling out for help, I turned the TV up so loud it woke the whole floor. The pandemonium brought attention and, at last, a trip to the bathroom. The annoyed nurse showed me the correct call button, which was on a different control pad on a table across the room.

This time, I decided to undo my boots and go to the bathroom alone. It takes too long for an answer to the call button, and these IV drips make my "back teeth float." I know I'm the world's worst patient and understand that nurses are overworked, but I would highly recommend that if you stay overnight, have someone stay with you. Either hire a private nurse for the night or have a cot brought into the room for a family member or friend. Most accidents and deaths in hospitals happen at night.

Mom used to love sharing nursing stories, but they've changed — and not for the better. She once said, "Gone are the days when a nurse could really be a nurse and give patients soothing back rubs. Now we run from room to room, fill out paperwork, and barely have time to do the basics."

I'd have loved a backrub right then. Hell, I'd just like to have used the bathroom.

My shining light last night was a phone call from Peter's cousin Arty. Talking was difficult because my throat was sore from the breathing tube during surgery and from the vomiting afterward. Last year Arty was diagnosed with thyroid cancer and multiple lymph-node invasions. After his operation he was quarantined for radiation treatments that involved drinking radioactive cocktails delivered by nurses in space suits.

Even his urine was checked with a Geiger counter to measure radio-activity. That is *waaay* scarier than anything I've gone through. Arty is fine now and reassures me that I will be, too. I needed to hear that.

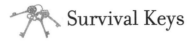 ## Survival Keys

* Seek out triumphant stories, they are important to anyone going through a life trauma.

* Learn from others how to survive. We learn from each other how to survive.

* Know that you are not alone. This is one of the things you will learn by sharing your emotions and challenges.

Chapter 10

THE WANNABE DOCTOR FROM HELL

*Intuitive aspects of healing means connecting with your physician
within to combine conventional and holistic medicine that
creates a healing that is greater than the sum of its individual parts.*
— Kathleen O'Keefe-Kanavos

♥ **Affirmation:** I will embrace pain and burn it as fuel for my healing journey.

At 5:30 a.m. a nurse pins a pink ribbon on the sleeve of my sore arm to alert medical personnel not to use it for taking my blood pressure. What a great idea! Then she gently places my arm on a small pillow and says, "There, that'll feel better." I wish she'd been here the prior night. Medical students knock and call out my name softly as they come in, turning on the overhead light. They empty the drain below my armpit and peer at my incision. It's nice to see so many female medical students. I felt their healing power even before I saw them.

"Perhaps the reason you are so nauseated is because of a link between breast surgery and nausea. Breast surgery stimulates hormones," one of the students says as she strokes my back during another nausea attack that brings a nurse in from the hallway to stroke the other side of my back. I guess I'm forgiven for last night's TV episode. I hold on to my incision area so my stitches won't tear while I vomit *and* balance a little barf bucket on my knees. After the attack passes, I lie back and cradle my painful breast. Can things get any worse? "Please don't bring that breakfast tray in here," I hear my voice say to someone in the doorway.

It's 6:30 a.m., and the medical student from hell enters my room. This young pipsqueak of a wannabe doctor flings open the door, flips on the overhead light, and yells across the room, "Ms. O'Keefe-Kanavos?"

I almost pee the bed as I sit up, yanking the drain in my back. The pain shocks me into full consciousness.

"What?" I yell back, sure there is an emergency in the building — fire, flood, or bomb!

"You look like you have a heart condition," Dr. Wannabe says, placing a stethoscope on my chest. Four students watched from behind him. I curled on my side trying not to puke again.

"I should say so, you nitwit," I growl, snatching the stethoscope from his ears and handing it back to him. "You almost gave me a heart attack by shocking me out of a sound sleep like that. I thought there was an emergency. Get out of my room, now!"

"You should watch your heart," Dr. Wannabe replies, appearing unfazed as he turns on his heels, dangling stethoscope in hand, flips off the light and promptly leaves the room, his minions close behind.

The good news is that my nausea has passed or I'd have barfed on him. My heart rate and temper are finally under control when another student nurse arrives.

"Take this," she orders with a smile, handing me a tiny white pill in a small white cup.

"What is it and what's it for?" I ask.

"It's insulin for your diabetes," she answers with a bigger smile.

"I don't have diabetes," I answered with no smile. "You're in the wrong room."

"Oh? Let me see your wrist, please." The smile vanishes as she plucks the little cup from my hand and makes a hasty exit. I just learned life lesson #5: Always ask, "What is that and what is it for?" concerning any medication given in the hospital. How do people survive here who are alone and can't ask these questions? This place is crazy.

It's time to go home, and my right hip has just erupted in sore, itchy shingles. I first got shingles at the university in Kentucky when bitten by a spider. Apparently, the spider had fallen out of a tree. Although my garments soaked up some of the venom, I still got a good dose, and in times of extreme stress, shingles appear. This is one of those times. I don't want Peter to tell the doctors about them because I don't want to be given medications that could have side effects or delay my treatments, and I don't want to have to stay another night here wearing these insufferable booties. Home will be a better place to heal in peace and quiet and with Baby Cakes for a nurse. At least he comes when I call.

One thing that gets rid of my shingles is kombucha tea brewed from mushrooms given to me by Jeanne from Virginia Beach. Peter brings some of the tea when he comes to pick me up. Taking it at hourly intervals gets the itchy tingle to stop.

After five days with Peter, Baby Cakes, Emergen-C, soaking in a shallow bath (mustn't get my incision wet), and kombucha tea, my shingles are gone. It always helps when the full moon smiles down on me through the skylight. "Didn't I just see you? Is it my imagination or are you checking up on me?" Thanks for checking on me," I tell the moon. "Hi, Mom. Love you."

Peter's head appears at the sound of my voice. "Bunny, who are you talking to?"

"Just Mom-in-the-moon."

Four days later I'm back in life-and-death reality. Finally! It's the big day of my final-final pathology report, and I'm jumping out of my skin while seated in Dr. Kritchen's waiting room. I want to know, but I don't want to know. Waiting for this report is just as difficult as waiting for the previous final pathology report had been. It doesn't get easier with time or practice. Again, my heart races while my body parts twitch. Where is that caterpillar with the hookah when I need it? And once more my report card from the University of Hard Knocks is good news/bad news.

Cancer was found in one lymph node, so all the lymph nodes were removed from my right armpit. No wonder I'm so swollen, sore, and blue — not just black and blue but literally blue from a dye used to check the sentinel node. Dr. Kritchen adds insult to injury when he tells me that I may never be able to play tennis or lift weights with my right arm again because of a condition called lymphedema, a swelling of the arm. Tennis is my way of making friends. Right now I really need some friends. I'm discouraged. My whole life is changing. Will anything ever be the same? Is there life after tennis? Is there life after crisis? If I hadn't convinced Dr. Wagner to operate on that invisible "hard spot," would I even have a life at all? When I ponder life after death, life after tennis doesn't seem so bad.

Two days after surgery, I started sleeping with my arm over my head and walking the wall with my fingers to exercise my muscles and teach my arm to find a way to get rid of the fluid buildup. To walk the wall, face it an arm's length away and walk your fingers up it as high as possible without undue pain. The rule is: if it hurts, *stop!* The swelling has gone down, and each day I can walk higher, so maybe I can still play tennis. Mind over matter!

As Dr. Kritchen tries to locate a printout in my ever-growing folder, I escape another anxiety attack by shutting my eyes to everything around me. My memory wanders back to Florida's subtropical ocean breezes and happier, healthier times. Peter and I are sitting on our dock, feet dangling over the water while we share a glass of wine at sunset. Pink clouds swirl in a hypnotic circular motion and silently explode with a display of heat lightning. We gaze up through the eye of a gigantic tornado that had begun its deadly descent to earth. It points like a finger at unsuspecting victims. We are lucky this day. The tornado passes over our home and hits a tiny city slightly north of us, practically wiping it off the map.

Today I'm gazing into the eye of an even deadlier storm. Can we be spared damage a second time as this tornado of trauma swirls above our heads, or will it touch down? Damn it! Even in my happy memories, I can't get away from my scary present. Will I ever get my emotions and mind back? I compare everything in my past life to my present crisis. I know that's not good but it's true. Cancer is like a tornado with no rhyme or reason to its path of destruction. It hits one family, jumps over two generations, and hits again without warning. All you have to do to get hit is be living.

Dr. Kritchen's voice draws me back the examining room. No warm breezes here, just ice-cold air conditioning. The good news? My margins were clean. Dr. Wagner has removed the entire cancerous area plus some healthy tissue despite his assumption that the tumor was not cancerous. A stroke of luck? Maybe my guides were talking in his ear, too. The report also states that the tumor cells are hormone receptive to estrogen. Therefore, he says, I will take the drug Tamoxifen for five years as one of my treatments after chemotherapy. Tamoxifen is a selective estrogen receptor modulator (SERM), and mimics estrogen by binding to estrogen receptors in the body, blah, blah, blah. What does this mean? Tamoxifen tricks receptors into not giving cells the order to multiply. I need all the tricks I can get.

My final pathology report: primary tumor 2.2 cm; invasive ducal carcinoma. The bad news? Rather than stage 1, stage-2 cancer with one node invaded.

Despite all the scary terms, Dr. Kritchen considers this an excellent prognosis and says so as he removes the drain from my back without pain. This report is really the first definitive good news we've gotten. I won't have to have my breast removed. The tumor is bigger than we originally thought, and a lymph node was invaded, but all in all it's better than it might have been, at least that's what I keep telling myself. I don't hear any voices disagree.

"How soon can I start chemo?" I ask Dr. Kritchen. The memory of the blood in the syringe still worries me.

"As soon as you get the okay from your oncologist."

My appointment with an oncologist is made for the next day, and I'm anxious to get started. I want to make sure nothing holds things up, like healing from surgery. I have this nagging desire to move things along. The clock is ticking. "I'm late, I'm late," I hear the white rabbit in my head pant.

As soon as Dr. Kritchen finishes his explanation of how treatable my cancer is and that he expects a full recovery, Peter walks outside the office, sits on the floor of the hallway, and, unfazed by the stares of the bustling crowd, cries like a baby. He cries so hard that he can't answer his cell phone. I think he's crying from all the stress we've experienced these past weeks, but through his sobs he explains that he's crying for joy. *Crying for joy?* I sit on the floor beside Peter, rock him, and find comfort in the realization that I will live. I guess this is a joyful moment, and this realization brings tears to my eyes. I'm glad I postponed my suicidal flight plan because it seems it will not be needed after all. I imagine the coroner looking over my exposed body and asking, "Why did she commit suicide? She could have beaten this."

With only minimal wind damage, we have once again looked a monster storm in the eye and were passed over. Life is full of storms, and I'm sure there will be plenty more on the horizon, because that is the nature of the beast called life crisis. The only way you can deal with a storm of this magnitude is one moment at a time, if necessary while seated in a busy medical hallway, crying for joy at having been diagnosed with stage-2 cancer. Crisis management.

Rocking back and forth with Peter, I fully appreciate what Dad went through when Mom was given her death sentence. The storm didn't pass over them. Now, I not only feel sympathy with their predicament but can also empathize with it. I've learned another difficult lesson at UHK: the difference between empathy and sympathy, the pathos fraternal twins, siblings so similar yet distinctly different, who were nurtured in the womb of Mother Compassion and delivered by Dr. Crisis. Empathy reaches for a deeper understanding through the experience of walking a mile in someone else's shoes, thereby feeling the pain, while Sister Sympathy understands how a person feels but does not share the depth of emotions because of a lack of personal or physical experience. Well, I now have empathy and sympathy in my emotional repertoire. This is called baptism by fire. I'm sure it's only the first of many lessons I'll learn in the near future.

As Peter and I collect ourselves emotionally and physically off the floor, Dr. Kritchen walks past with his ever-present Cheshire cat smile that disappears around the corner. If a caterpillar smoking a hookah crawls up next to me and asks, "Whooo are yooou?" It damned well better have some potent pieces of mushroom to share, because right now I could really use some help. I'd rather have a double martini, but the pipe will do as a second choice.

On the way home we phone family and friends with facts and

good news to balance out the bad. I had already called my sister-in law, because she is a ten-year breast cancer survivor. I knew she would understand our angst and need for support as only another survivor can. Being told you have cancer is like being called up to war then explaining your battle fears to someone who has never been out of the neighborhood. You need a veteran. My sister-in-law is that cancer war veteran. She can understand and sympathize with me, sisters in arms.

I've decided not to tell Dad about my condition because he just went through hell with Mom's death. It was too difficult for him to live in a home he and Mom had shared for twenty years, so he packed up and moved. Dad is adjusting nicely, and we didn't want to rock his boat. I'll tell him after my treatment is complete.

I hope my results come back from Dr. Nagourney before my first meeting with the oncologist to determine the course of treatment. My surgery site has healed well, so all in all things have improved; yet I'm still frightened. Is that normal? When does the fear subside?

 ## Survival Keys

* Face fear. The greatest fear is the fear of fear itself and is often a result of the unknown. Life is full of the unknown. Find the silver lining.

* Trust in the Law of Life that states, "Everything ends." Anyone going through any life trauma often wonders where and when the roller-coaster ride of uncertainty will end.

* Pray. Faith in a Higher Power can give comfort during dark hours. Prayer has power, and prayers can be answered in dreams.

* Keep a journal.

* Let go. Sometimes you must let God lead the way. She has wide shoulders.

Part II

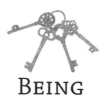

Being

Chapter 11

CALLING DR. CHEMO/DR. SPIDER

Joking is undignified; that is why it is so good for one's soul.
— G. K. Chesterton (1874–1936)

♥ *Affirmation:* I am my own unique self — special, creative, and wonderful.

Dr. Barkley, my oncologist, is the picture-perfect proper Bostonian, with a multicolored vest and neat little bow tie beneath his white medical coat. He holds you with his blue eyes as he scoots his delicately thin body around the examining room on a tiny four-wheeled black stool. This makes him look like a happy multicolored spider.

"You have a choice of two different chemotherapies and possibly another, called Taxol, at the end of your treatment, but we'll discuss that later," Dr. Barkley, says. "Adriamycin/Cytoxin, is a very aggressive treatment that involves four sessions over a three-month period, and you will lose all of your hair. The second choice is CMF, Cyclosphamide, Methotrexate, and Fluorouracil 5 FU; a six-month chemo of twelve treatments, one every two weeks, which will cause you to lose twenty to forty percent of your hair." He wheels over and gazes up to where I sit on the papered examining table.

I think of how I read food labels and do not eat anything I can't pronounce. Now I'm going to have similarly unknown ingredients go into my veins. How often do I take the six-month one? My brain feels like it has shut down and I can't seem to hear. I think I'm experiencing hysterical deafness again. I'm thankful Peter is here to repeat this. My doctor is waiting for an answer. I can't remember the question. I'm saved by a knock at the door.

In a quiet voice that I can hear, a nurse says, "A doctor from California just faxed over this information concerning Kathleen's chemotherapy treatment and is waiting on the phone to speak with you." I can hear her whispering across the room, but I can't hear the doctor speaking right to me. What's wrong with this picture? The doctor on the phone must be Dr. Nagourney from California with my CSRA test results. This is incredible synchronicity.

Dr. Barkley calls over his shoulder, "Think about the treatments. I'll be right back."

Peter and I look at each other. "What a choice," I moan and cover my face with my hands. "And I can't even remember what they are." Peter slowly repeats them. The longer I listen, the more upset I become. The way I see it, my choices are a bald head for a short time or scraggly hair for half a year. Three months or six months? Six months is too long. I want to get back to my life. I swing my feet back and forth to calm myself. My predicament reminds me of a joke that isn't funny right now but fits the situation: Death by Roo-Roo.

Two missionaries are captured by warriors in a jungle and taken before the chief who informs them they have a choice of two punishments for trespassing. "The first punishment is to be taken into the jungle where all my warriors will sexually have their way with you. This is called Roo-Roo. The second is death!" The first missionary quickly answers, "I'll take Roo-Roo." The second missionary thinks for a second and says, "I'll take death."

"Take the first missionary into the jungle for Roo-Roo," replies the chief, "and the second one into the jungle for death by Roo-Roo."

A joke I had always thought so funny suddenly has new meaning. I begin to cry. But when Dr. Barkley returns, I'm composed; my decision has been validated by the report from Dr. Nagourney. Only one chemotherapy treatment killed the tumor: Adriamycin Cytoxin, AKA AC, the Purple Death. In fact, the doctor in California asked if I had

had chemotherapy before, because my tissue's resistance to the drugs had been so high. Anyway, I've chosen to be baldheaded with four treatments of Roo-Roo.

"When can I start my chemo?"

"How about Thursday, the day after tomorrow?"

With my course of treatment so final and my hair loss only two days away, I break down and cry so hard the doctor and his nurse leave the office to give us space to come to terms with our decision. I say "our decision" because Peter has been an active part of this whole process and now he's crying as hard as I am. The thought of giving up my long hair, even for a short time, devastates me.

I peer up at Peter through raccoon eyes of smeared mascara and declare, "Demi Moore looked great in the movie GI Jane, and she chose to shave her head. If she could survive being bald, then I can, too."

On our way out of the hospital, while trying to dry tears that wouldn't stop, Peter says, "Look, here's a wig shop for cancer patients. Let's see what they have." It's the Friends Boutique on the oncology floor. I'd noticed it earlier but hurried past, sure that treatment had improved so patients no longer had to deal with baldness, which seemed to add insult to injury. No such luck. I'll come to terms with wigs later — but not today. Today, I'm done dealing. In fact I want nothing to do with "that place" and make this perfectly clear to Peter as I watch the elevator doors close on him mid-sentence. "But they may —" Ten minutes later he exited into the lobby with brochures in his hand and a smile on his face. I greeted him with "Don't even hand those to me." He tucked them into his jacket pocket, out of sight but not out of mind. We walked to the car in awkward silence. *I've hit saturation point, I'm angry, frightened, and sad.* LEAVE ME ALONE!

This morning, as we breakfast in our sunny dining room, Peter and I speak about how we'll get through all of this together. He feels such guilt because for so long I was not number one in his life, and it was difficult for me. As an only child of my parents' second marriage, I'm used to being number one. Tommy, my half brother, was nineteen when I was born. He joined the army two years later. My family's pecking order was obvious: Daddy Bear, Momma Bear, and the apple of their eye, Baby Bear. Peter's Greek family, especially after his father's death, depended on him as if he were the head of the family because he was the eldest, so he became Daddy Bear of a very large bear clan whose pecking order had gone through a radical change. Their needs came first. The family business came second. My husband came third, and I fourth. When and why did I give up being number one? That's a good question. Let me think about that for a moment. I think the answer will be cathartic....

It happened so gradually that I didn't notice the shift in order until it was complete. But I allowed it to happen and must take responsibility for that. I've never had a victim mentality; I've always believed that you can't be victimized without your permission. Unwittingly, naively, through passive acquiescence, I gave that permission. However, I'm not sure that I would have done things differently if I'd known then what I know now, because I'm the type of person who trusts people until they prove that they're untrustworthy, especially family.

It was right after Peter's father died and his family was sent into a tailspin that I gave up my position. Peter's father was larger than life, and I felt I was strong enough to take a back seat to his family until they got back on their feet and adjusted to their new situation. Well, some of them never wanted to give up the front seat once they settled into it. That was one of the reasons Peter and I decided to move to Cape Cod: to become autonomous again and slowly give up the family business. My acquiescing to this back-seat arrangement was the perfect example of that old saying "No good deed goes unpunished." But guilt has very long arms and can reach across time and space to hold tight to old habits and expectations. My friends, in whom I confided, told me this problem was a "Greek thing" and an expected part of marrying into that culture. I didn't agree. I think it's an insecurity thing, experienced by needy people frightened by change. When I stepped aside, I gave up my power as wife.

Social pecking orders are interesting. I experienced them frequently as an army brat. There were two ways to position yourself into a new pecking order: fight or look for an old friend to help you cut in line. Whenever possible, I chose the peaceful route.

There is another old saying: "You can choose your friends but not your family." I don't agree with that either. Toxic fruit can grow on family trees. Once you're old enough to choose your life, you're old enough to choose your family or what you choose to keep of it.

Well, I've come to the conclusion that riding in the back seat makes me carsick, so I must be number one again. It's unfortunate that it has come down to them or me. I was there for them. Now it's time for me.

So today, in the dining room, Peter and I vow that from now on I am his "number one" and he is mine. No one and nothing will come before or between us. We hold hands in our bathrobes and cry as it begins to snow in the full sunshine. The golden flakes are so beautiful that we stand outside in the cold, in our robes, and promise to love each other forever and get through this ordeal day by day as we change our lives for the better.

Peter says he has told his family that he will not work away from the house during my crisis but will work as much as he can from home. Most of them understand. This will be a challenge for those who don't, but I believe challenges result in spiritual and emotional growth — the larger the challenge the bigger the growth. We are all going to be emotionally bigger after this is all over. And those who aren't would probably never have been, anyway, but this is not my problem anymore.

It's time for my next step: find a wig close to my own hair color and style before I lose it and forget what it looks like. While I go through all this "stuff" I still want to look like me. Most of all I want to look healthy, and then I can catch up to my looks and be healthy.

Here are some facts and figures from the national Alopecia Areata Foundation to help during your hair crisis:

* In the U.S., 4.5 million men, women, and children suffer from hair loss, or alopecia. (We're not alone.)

* Stress is often a cause. Hair usually grows back under normal circumstances, but since there are no norms (rule #4), there are treatments available to stimulate regrowth.

* Over 30 million women have some kind of baldness, causing them to lose sight of who they are.

Well, I'm counting on my hair growing back after treatment, but in case it doesn't, I'll file this information away for future use and pray I don't need it. Now, I must prepare myself physically, mentally, and emotionally for chemotherapy.

 ## Survival Keys

* Focus on your essence. Your essence is not about your hair, breasts, uterus, or other physical attributes.

* Take time to look inward. Your essence is what is inside you.

* Embrace your emotions. It is rational to be emotional during a crisis. Embrace your emotions, but don't let them rule you.

Chapter 12
NO PAIN, NO GAIN

To deal effectively with a crisis, we must get in touch with
our inner selves and work together toward the goal of survival.
— Kathleen O'Keefe-Kanavos

♥ *Affirmation:* I will use humor as another defense against trauma
in my universe.

My first day of chemotherapy is not good. We arrive late because of
an unexpected snowstorm. My cell-phone call to warn the nurses was
tossed around the automated phone system for what felt like forever,
then ended up back where it began — on hold. I gave up and told the
front-desk secretary what had happened, forty-five minutes later.

"Oh, that happens to everyone when they get into the automated
hospital phone system." She handed me a small card. "Next time dial
this number; it'll ring through to our desk."

Despite her smile, I was cranky. No doubt it was related to my fear
of the unknown. I had no idea what I was in for today and was afraid
to find out. Hopefully, the nurse was used to this sort of thing and
wouldn't take my puss-face personally. (These people deserve med-
als.) I finally make it to Dr. Barkley's office and discover I'd just started
what he tells me will probably be my last menstrual cycle. With an
apologetic look he explains that chemotherapy will put me into early
menopause — "No more periods."

Does this mean that I can wear white pants whenever and wher-
ever I want, even on long vacations? When I empty my purse in restaurants to find my keys, I won't have tampons fall out all over the

71

place? And what about bloating, cramps, heating pads, and Midol? Will I have to live without them, too? I think I'll throw a party. What a great side effect!

Dr. Barkley pointed out another chemotherapy side effect: mouth sores. No party there. He suggested that during treatment I wash my mouth out only with warm salt water and not brush my teeth because that can stir up bacteria and cause bigger problems, such as septice-mia — infection in the bloodstream. "And don't use mouthwash or other products with alcohol because they'll only dry out your mouth more and cause complications."

Great! Don't brush my teeth and they might fall out, or brush my teeth and they might fall out. Sounds like death by Roo-Roo. I need a double martini — oh — no alcohol. This sucks.

Time for more fun: up to the tenth floor for a blood test, then back down to the ninth floor for my first chemo session. I beg the nurse to leave the needle in so I won't have to be stuck a second time for chemo, but she said my infusion nurse would do her own insertion.

Don't they realize that some patients have only one arm to work with and only a few veins left in that arm? I hope my veins hold up. I hope my temper holds up. They need to rethink this rule, so I decide I'll *share* this insight with the doctor on my next visit. No doubt he'll be thrilled with my opinion, but if enough people complain maybe the rule will be changed in favor of the patient. "Deep breaths, Kathy," I whisper as I follow the nurse to the infusion chair.

After five attempts to get my vein, the IV nurse gives up and calls a psychiatrist who deals in pain control. I guess I looked out of con-trol when I curled up in a ball with my arm safely tucked away and refused to let anyone touch me. Then I turn into a real bitch and tell the nurses to go to the basement of the Brigham and Women's Hospital and look for any Asian men in blue surgical scrubs. "They're Chinese, not Japanese, so don't insult them. They'll know what they're doing." I also told them that if they couldn't find someone Chinese, to just grab me a doctor, any doctor. I was very serious. They were not amused. Peter tried his best to comfort me but didn't know what to do, so he brought me tea.

When the psychiatrist/pain specialist arrives, I'm moved to a dark room. We chat for a few minutes and her soft voice quiets my inner warrior. Then she calls in one of the best IV nurses on the floor who peers at my arm, then at me, wraps my arm in hot towels, gives me an Ativan, and leaves. Ativan is similar to Valium. Twenty minutes later she returns and is successful at finding a vein that will not blow up, roll away, or hide.

Nurse Deana looks slightly amused when I ask her if she will be my IV nurse from now on. She says she'll ask the floor supervisor for permission.

I'm so happy. It pays to be your own advocate, because Doreen, the head nurse/floor supervisor, informs me that I can have Deana each time I come. I don't know how happy Deana will be about this, because I don't think anyone else wants me. The pain-control specialist will return on my next appointment to make sure things go well. I feel a little more in control because the problem of my veins has been solved and I have someone to watch over me. There is a tiny light at the end of this dark and scary tunnel called treatment.

With my IV needle comfortably in place, Deana hooks me up to a bag of hydrating solution before she administers the chemotherapy. I didn't realize how important these nausea and hydration medications are until a friend told me a frightening story about the sister of a tennis friend who went through this same chemo. She had become very dehydrated from vomiting after treatment. Her husband traveled for work so she was home alone. One night she couldn't stop vomiting and called a neighbor to take her to the hospital. The friend took her to a nearby emergency room rather than the one where she went for her treatments. (This story does not have a happy ending, so if you are going through this for the first time, skip to the next paragraph and hand this part to your caregiver. I've included it because it's an important lesson that could save a life.) The personnel in the emergency room didn't have the experience or training to deal with chemotherapy dehydration, so they put a tube down her throat for liquids and left her alone. She choked to death on her vomit. Her family was devastated and her husband filled with guilt. The lesson is: Cancer centers know how to deal with treatment problems. Keep their number handy and call them if you need help.

My chemotherapy, Adriamycin and Cytoxan (A/C), looks like grape Kool-Aid and is given as a push rather than as a drip from a bag. Deana explained that A/C can seriously irritate tissue if any of the liquid escapes onto or into the skin.

A/C may also turn my fingernails dark. (Lovely! Can't wait!) Well, if they're dark enough I won't have to wear nail polish, and if they aren't dark enough there's always Chanel's Vamp or other popular Goth colors. But the best part is my urine is the same Kool-Aid color. Yeah! Talk about an eye opener. I wonder what this is doing to my kidneys and bladder, but dismiss the thought as too scary to contemplate. I'm so wigged out by the grape-colored urine that I drink extra cups of water. When the doctors or nurses see me wheeling my hanging IV bags toward the bathroom with a look of fixed determination on my face, they get out of the way. They don't want to be IV roadkill.

After one such bathroom run, Dr. Barkley magically appears next to my infusion chair to explain my chemotherapy regimen. He also shares more good news: I must go to the Cape Cod Hospital weekly and have blood drawn for analysis. That is just what I need to hear right now after the fiasco I went through this morning. But I use this opportunity to segue into the suggestion of using only one needle on infusion days. He is sympathetic but explains, "This is hospital policy. You could have a port (short for portable catheter) surgically placed in your chest area. Then your chemo is hooked right into the port."

I'm not a big fan of scars. I had asked women in the elevators about their ports. I'm no longer shy and have learned to ask the other guinea pigs. They possess a wealth of knowledge from experience and are usually more than happy to share information. Most of the ports I've seen, and the one Dr. Barkley suggested, are one-way ports. They aren't used to take blood out, only to put chemo in. That reinforces my decision to pass on the port idea. I have a better idea: ONLY USE ONE $#%& NEEDLE! Hospital policies do not seem to be patient friendly or logical.

The whole infusion process took five hours, and on the drive home I'm completely wiped out and sleep — until I have to go to the bathroom again. Poor Peter had to make gas station and McDonalds restaurant pit stops. The good news? No more Kool-Aid pee-pee.

Earlier today Dr. Barkley explained that the side effects would be cumulative; each treatment would make me weaker and sicker. Deana gave me a list of times to take my anti-nausea drugs. It seems like an awful lot of pills, but after my tennis friend's story, I don't want to get nauseated and die alone. I wonder how I'll feel tomorrow.

Someone please shoot me. I'd shoot myself but I've lost all my strength. I can't lift my head, let alone a weapon. Fortunately I haven't lost my sense of humor yet. I can't make it out of bed, and it's only the first day after treatment. Oh, my God! What have I gotten myself into? Is this normal? I've got a bad case of the hiccups — an early warning barf symptom. I get them when it's time for my anti-nausea medication. I've taken baths twice a day because my joints, muscles, and back hurt so badly. Thank goodness this chemo is only three months long. I couldn't take six months.

I absolutely must brush my teeth after I puke, and have devised a plan of dipping floss into hydrogen peroxide and then brush with Rembrandt toothpaste mixed with hydrogen peroxide, followed by a rinse called H.P.M. (Hydrogen Peroxide Mouthwash) from the health food store. This has to be better than not brushing for three months.

My oncologist's concern about dangerous bacteria in the mouth during treatment is understandable; however, research in the *New England Journal of Medicine* reveals that the presence of periodontal disease doubles your risk of heart attack. Yeah, that's all I need on top of everything else: survive cancer to die of a heart attack for not brushing my teeth during treatment. More death by Roo-Roo. Well, it would be a quicker death. Reading these articles brings back memories of dinner discussions, memories I'd stored in the back of my mind for future use. I guess the future is now.

I remember a talk with Dad after one of his Green Beret six-month disappearing acts, the result of an early morning "Red Alert."

He never told us where he'd been but spoke of the Middle Eastern women brought to his Special Forces MASH Unit. They had such advanced periodontal disease that all the doctors could do was give them Vitamin C tablets and send them home to die. I couldn't have realized then how important that conversation would be now.

Something unusual happened tonight: The sound of horses' hooves and buggy wheels on our driveway woke me. I dragged myself from bed and followed the sounds to the front door. Peter came out of the TV room and asked where I was going. We opened the door and looked out. Nothing was there. The sounds had stopped. As I climbed back into bed I wondered who had just arrived, how long they planned to stay, and if they'd be quieter than the soldier-spirits in Berlin.

It's been three days since my first chemotherapy, and I've come to an important conclusion: I don't want to ever look back at this time in my life. I will burn these journals at the end of my treatment. The only reflection I want to study is my healthy one in the mirror. I only want to look *forward* to a time of plenty, plenty of luncheons, tennis, dancing, scuba diving, and *health. No more illness or voices. Do you hear me?* If I've learned one thing during this ordeal, it's that being sick sucks!

I feel so alone and lost in my feelings. Where is my support system? Mom is dead. My friends and Dad are in Florida. I think I need to talk to a professional.

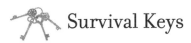 Survival Keys

✳ Get professional help. Feelings of isolation and fear are normal reactions to crisis, but that doesn't make them any less important. Conversations with and guidance from professionals can help promote successful growth from traumatic experiences.

✳ Make healthy changes. By pointing out unhealthy life and emotional patterns that are contributing factors to the crisis, healthy changes can be made.

✳ Don't travel alone. No one has to travel the road of trauma alone. If your doctors request counseling for you, some insurance companies will pay for the sessions.

Chapter 13

SOMEONE TO TALK TO

We are all droplets of light from the Ocean of Gnosis
that have descended onto the earth plane. By being
of service we become enlightened.
— Kathleen O'Keefe-Kanavos

♥ *Affirmation:* I am safe to express my needs and wants. I now
attract only joyful relationships.

I don't need psychotherapy. I know crazy, and I'm not there — not
yet. But there are some things I feel comfortable discussing only with
another woman. I need space and a friend. I need someone to talk to.

My brother in-law phones to check on me and offers the phone
number of friends of his. "Roger's wife has been going through cancer
for seven years and would gladly speak with you," he says. Seven years.
What bad luck! They must have broken a really big mirror. I need
someone to talk to but not someone stuck in Cancerland for seven
years. We'd have nothing in common, because when I'm finished with
treatment, I'm NOT coming back to this nightmare.

As unified as Peter and I are, there are things that I don't want to
share with him because I think he is suffering from sympathy pains.
He has enough on his plate ... me. He says he understands my need to
talk with someone and that there is a holistic center down the street.
He calls and speaks with a therapist who agrees to see me. I'm still
too woozy from all the drugs to navigate a car on these ocean roads,
so Peter drives.

The therapist introduces herself as Linda and hands me her card, which features the face of a wolf. She looks like an old hippie with long gray hair parted in the middle and an ankle-length, multi-print flowing dress and socks with sandals — in the dead of winter. The sunlit room was filled with potted plants beneath windows that face the water. Did she come to work in those sandals? My eyes pause on an old pair of well-loved Ugg-type boots with rundown heels leaning against the wall in the corner. "I was a wolf in a previous life," she explains, drawing my attention back to her. She continues with "Then I was an Indian."

Okay. Either she needs therapy, too, or I'm in the right place. I'll decide later.

Linda wanted to meet with both of us first, so we sit in identical chairs and explain our situation to the hippie therapist. She listens intently, then abruptly says to Peter, "I'd like to speak to Kathy alone now. If you want a therapist, you'll need to find your own."

Peter looks surprised but says okay. He closes the door quietly behind him on his way out to the waiting room. My shock turns to agreement when I remember an article Peter had shown me two days ago: "The Ten Leading Stresses For Heart Attacks: Do You Have One?" Peter had seven of the ten. He qualifies for his own therapist.

"Now," Linda says, moving her chair closer to mine while handing me a box of tissues, "start from the beginning and tell me everything." So I did — what I had experienced emotionally and physically, and how I'm not only grieving for the loss of my mother but also for myself. My innocence has died and now I'm worried that my body might follow.

"Having a passive wish to join a loved one is part of the grieving process and one of the healing steps. Attempting suicide to join that person changes normal into what is known as complicated grief, which can often be helped with medication. Are you thinking of suicide?" she asks gently.

I remember my thoughts during the "hour of souls" and give an honest answer. "No, but I wonder if my body is. I was close to my mother, but never thought I was so close that I'd want to join her. We all have to die someday, but I really don't want to die yet."

"Good. I think you are simultaneously experiencing a number of losses. Tell me how many of these causes of grief pertain to you right now: The death of a loved one, miscarriage, pet loss, major life change, and anticipation of a loss such as a diagnosis of a terminal illness."

Well, I didn't need to think long. Bluey, my sixteen-year-old Siamese cat, had died in my arms six months prior. Grief stricken, I couldn't get out of bed for days, so the only loss from the list that didn't fit my life right now was miscarriage. The memory of Dr. Barkley's belated warning, "be sure to use protection during sex with your treatments because you could still get pregnant," reminds me that that could change, too. The other three causes of grief fit me on multiple levels, and I tell this to Linda. It feels odd being reminded of the signs of grief rather than reminding someone else of them. Now I'm the client rather than the therapist or the psychology professor. The tables are turned, and the twin professors, Empathy and Sympathy, from the University of Hard Knocks, are not holding back on my lessons.

Linda looks down at her sandaled feet for a second and then says with all seriousness, "You certainly have grounds to grieve, and you are in crisis. Now let's go over the steps and see where you are." She must have dealt with a lot of bereavement because she recites the five steps without even blinking: "Denial of loss, anger, yearning, despair, acceptance of loss."

"Well, I'm past the first two concerning my mother and my diagnosis. I still yearn for my mother and for my healthy life. I was angry with my doctors for not listening to me, but I realize they were just following hospital policy. That caused me despair. But I've accepted Mom's death and my predicament, which is step five, so you tell me where that leaves me. Am I stuck somewhere in the middle and no longer progressing, or did I just skip over the middle to the end?"

"I think you are going through a very difficult time and progressing very well. But how do you feel you're doing? How does having all this come at you at once make you feel?"

"Well, sometimes I feel like life is beating me down and every time I try to get up it yells, "Stay down! Cry uncle!" But I can't give up or cry uncle."

"Why not?"

"Because it goes against my nature, my inner warrior and the fighting Irish in me. I'm not a victim. I'm not even a victim of circumstances. I self-advocated and will continue to."

"Good! Now let's talk about your relationships."

She understands my concerns about previously not having been number one in Peter's life, and that though he has pledged his support to me, his family pulls at him harder than ever, even though they're aware of our crisis.

"Nothing is more important to them than themselves," she explains about Peter's family. "You will never change them, but you can change your response to them. Then they'll have to adjust to this new response."

She was absolutely right and confirmed what I had realized days earlier after a phone call from an angry family member that reduced Peter to tears. Basic Behavior Modification 101 states: The quickest way to change someone's behavior is to change yours first. Years of teaching Special Education taught me that before behavior gets better, it inevitably gets worse, and if you don't get the response you want, continue until you do. The key word here is "respond." Don't inadvertently *react* to their inappropriate behavior; consciously *respond* to it, even if that means ignoring it. Another life lesson from the past now being used in the present.

Linda says, "I'm going to give you a mantra to repeat to yourself whenever you don't feel like the most significant person in your life, because that is what you need to feel right now." She leans toward me in her chair and says, "I am number one. No one and nothing is more important than I. Repeat this mantra as often as you need until you start to feel it. If your husband can't come to terms with the fact that you need his full support and are his immediate family now, and that you need him more than his other family, who really need to grow up, you might need to make some permanent changes. He is from a Greek culture, and this antiquated way of thinking might be too ingrained in him to change."

She might be right, but I wasn't ready to throw in the towel on my marriage, and I certainly didn't want to let Peter's family break us up. Again, my fighting Irish stirred as my Xena, Warrior Princess honed her sword.

"Encourage Peter to seek therapy because he is facing some over-whelming issues, too. But right now your attention needs to be on yourself and not on him. Be selfish. His issues have to do with let-ting go of the past, his family, and growing up. You are his family now. His old family must either sink or swim. Peter can't swim for them anymore. No one can swim for someone else." She patted my hand. "I'll be here for you, and when you don't feel up to coming in, we can talk by phone."

I felt so much better. Linda was definitely a keeper, especially since she was part wolf and Indian. I'd dealt with Indian spirits in Virginia Beach, but never wolves. This would be a good experience.

Later that night Peter and I light candles in our bathroom, turn on soft classical music, and soak in the Jacuzzi just as we had the night this all began, so many months — lifetimes — ago. As we rub each other's feet, I answer some of Peter's questions about what the thera-pist said after he had left the room, mostly the part about finding his own therapist and why.

"If you want a divorce, I'll stay with you until you're well and make sure you're cared for the rest of your life," Peter says with tears in his eyes. "I know I haven't been a good husband, but I'll try to change. I feel guilty about all that has happened and about not having given you the attention you needed and deserved. I didn't realize how unhappy you were. You know I love you more than anything in this world." Large tears roll down his face and pop the bubbles in the water as they drop off his chin stubble. I feel badly for him. I know he's trying hard and that he had a long and rocky road to travel, both with my condition and his family. In a way, Peter too has lost his family as he knew it.

My husband was no stranger to cancer. His father had died of it, and Peter had watched me care for Mom before she died of it. Like me, Peter was afraid and shell shocked from all the cancer wars that had been fought and lost. The pain in his eyes explained the fears he couldn't voice. What could keep lightning from striking again?

To impress on him how much he meant to me and how much I loved him, I tell him a love story about how I fell in love with him.

When I was living in Florida, and thought I'd never find the right person to spend the rest of my life with, I had this little chat with God.

"Look," I said, after rejecting yet another date, "if there's someone you want me to be with the rest of my life, please bring him on. If I'm to stay single that's fine too, but please don't send me any more losers. What must I do to find the love of my life?"

A week later, on Sadie Hawkins Day, I met Peter in a grungy bar. A friend was having second thoughts about her impending divorce and had asked me to meet her for a drink and a chat. A private con·versation was difficult as chairs around our table filled with men who offered us booze, dances, and their screws. Yes, their screws. At the door, women were given bolts and men screws for the annual party, held on the first Saturday in November since 1938 by cartoonist Al Capp, who'd invented Sadie Hawkins Day for his *Li'l Abner* comic strip. Sadie Hawkins was the homely unwed daughter of the Mayor of Hillbilly Dogpatch who pursued the top eligible bachelors in a run-for-your-life footrace. The ultimate prize was matrimony for the spinsters. And here I was, single and at the party for the spinsters.

But the goal at this party was to find your partner by getting "screwed." I threw my bolt away after a Neanderthal's screw almost fit. Just when I thought I couldn't take anymore, in walked handsome Peter. He walked up to my table with all the confidence in the world and asked me to dance. I was instantly drawn to this gorgeous Greek with sun-streaked hair and the most beautiful soft brown eyes I'd ever seen. I fell in love through the windows to Peter's soul. We spent the next three years together until the day my in-laws gave us a society wedding at Copley Plaza in Boston. My father-in-law always said, "Kathy ran from Peter just fast enough to catch him." If Peter was my Li'l Abner, then I was his Daisy Mae. With Peter by my side, I felt God had answered my prayers. "Ask and ye shall receive" had worked. I tell Peter this now, while we rub each other's feet in the tub.

"I didn't want to be with anyone else on earth then, and I feel the same way now," I told him and caressed his pinky toe. "If we get divorced we might have bigger problems in our next marriages." We vowed never to let the "d" word, "divorce," come up again. We can work it out.

Just like the night Peter first found my invisible spot, this was another emotional, life-changing, sensual bubble bath. We seemed to accomplish a lot in the tub. I look up through our skylight to see Mom's full moon. God, I've gone through so many changes in such a short time my head spins thinking about them. Or is it the effects of the chemo and anti-nausea drugs compounded by a warm bath? While gazing at the moon, I'm struck by another lesson I've mastered: compassion. I've seen women in therapy comforted by husbands, and seen many alone. Peter is always with me. I'm so lucky not to have to go through this by myself; another silver lining discovered beneath the light of the silvery moon.

Maybe all this mental babble in the bubble bath is God saying, "I didn't send you a perfect man. I sent the perfect man for you. You took vows before me. When the priest blessed you, I blessed you with the sound of unscheduled cathedral bells. Now go and continue to grow together, and here's some extra cement to bind you together, 'cause you're gonna need it!"

Crisis affects the whole family. Life Lesson #6: Crisis challenges relationships. The closer the relationship the greater the challenge, because deep emotions result in big cracks. Troubles make relationships either grow stronger or fall apart, but they never stay the same.

Relationships are like bricks in an arch, two or more entities fused together to become one. When an earthquake such as trauma shakes those bonds to their foundation, cracks form. If relationship cracks are ignored, perhaps from denial, they grow larger until they split completely. But if relationship rifts are examined with soul searching and repaired with love and respect, the attachment can become so strong that when everything else is reduced to rubble, the arch survives.

When the Japanese mend broken objects, they enhance the damage by filling the cracks with gold in the belief that when something suffers damage it acquires a history and becomes more beautiful. John F. Kennedy summed up relationships in his address of 12 April 1959: "When written in Chinese, the word "crisis" is composed of two characters: one represents danger and the other represents opportunity."

Opposites do attract.

Survival Keys

✳ Find the golden nuggets in your dreams, meditations, and prayers and use them to mend the cracks in your relationships.

✳ Find the answers to enduring relationships. It is possible, even during crisis.

Chapter 14

My Head/My House: 4 Ways to Overcome Inner Chaos

Dreams are the phone line by which our Inner ET (Eternal Teacher) phones home. What is truly amazing is that the call is always answered by someone on the other side.

— Kathleen O'Keefe-Kanavos

♥ *Affirmation:* I choose to make positive healthy choices for myself.

The people in my head make up my total being necessary to fight and win in any crisis. I not only have an inner child, inner teenager, and inner adult — who would be equivalent to the id, ego, and superego — I have inner grandparents who are unafraid to express their opinions.

When first faced with crisis, my inner house went into a state of chaos and four things instantly happened:

Children ran up and down the halls yelling, "No hospitals, no needles, and no doctors!"

My teenagers slammed their doors and locked themselves in their rooms.

My parents wanted to have meetings, while the grandparents dug up every piece of emotional baggage they had ever buried, complete with the coulda-woulda-shouldas and the dreaded what-ifs.

I had to get my house under control and used these three steps with solutions.

The first step was to catch those kids. The best way to do that was to sing and get them to join in. Anything simple would do — *Mary Had*

86

a Little Lamb, the Mickey Mouse Club song — something so simple that they won't think scary thoughts.

The next step was coaxing the teenagers out of their rooms. Denial and sleep is their therapy of choice. To get them to attend an inner-house meeting led by the parents is a chore. To get the teenagers out of their rooms I give them a challenge: make the children sing by dancing for them. Teens love to dance! Music is magic.

To deal with grandparents, I use humor to get them to sit down and laugh, then the teenagers hold them in their rocking chairs while the children tie them up with jump ropes.

Everyone has an important purpose in the house within my mind.

Children bring primal emotion, spontaneity, laughter, and song.

Teenagers are incredible problem solvers. Tell them a square peg won't fit into a round hole, and they're off to find the saw and hammer. They know no limits, think they're immortal, and, face with danger-ous challenges, often suggest amazing solutions that work.

Parents determine which solutions are too dangerous to try, and grandparents remember why the solutions did or didn't work before.

That can be the basis for inner bliss or battles, because being at odds with self is self-defeating. United you stand, divided you fall. Dreams are the glue that can cement your family.

Billy is a developmentally disabled sixteen-year-old who lives in my inner house and often pops up in my dreams. Family members are very protective of Billy, particularly the teenagers, who often wrap their arms around him. He is important because his questions are truthful and direct, such as, "Why are you bald?" When someone answered, "Billy, we're all bald from the chemotherapy we agreed to take," he just smiled and rocked back and forth on the balls of his feet. I was actually too shocked to answer. *What a rude question*, I thought. But that's Billy's gift to our family — his directness can elicit a defensive response by its pure honesty. If I ask Billy, "Why are you doing that?" he'll grin and answer, "'Cause I need to." Honest and to the point. Billy is always happy and is the tallest person in the crowd of teenagers. Despite his low mental capacity he's heads above the rest.

Inner grandparents are sentimental pack rats and use emotions and memories to make decisions, reverently dragging them all out of their closets whenever the occasion warrants. They have memories like elephants and store everything that has ever happened to us in this and possibly past lives. Their suitcases bulge with experience. Crisis time is a reason to sort through it all again and again. "See, I told you so. This happened before. Now will you listen? We could have done that." This can go on for days if not stopped.

After a couple glasses of wine, the emotional pitch party begins: We pitch out all the old emotions attached to memories that no longer fit our lives. A crisis brings emotions into the open for discussion. How do I get the parents and grandparents to stop howling while we toss out their precious baggage? Give them a good riddle to think about and discuss! They love to discuss an issue or idea to death. I ask, "What if (their favorite phrase) the world were square? Would we all be SpongeBob SquarePants?" It works. I finally have piece of mind.

Here are three reasons to understand and embrace your inner family:

Inner family is reassuring because you are never alone, on many levels, even during your darkest hours. You're always with family who are friends and have your best interests at heart. This might seem like a case of too many chiefs and not enough Indians, but remember: you always have the final say.

Add you inner family's two cents to your spiritual guides' two cents and you'll be pretty darned rich.

To effectively deal with a crisis you must get in touch with your inner selves and work together toward the goal of survival. Do that every minute of every day by using you inner guidance in the form of dreams, meditation, and prayers.

Three months to the day after my birthday gift of a cancer-free mammogram, my hair with its chemo-blackened roots falls out by the handful, slides down the shower walls, and clogs the drain. Peter uses the toilet plunger to free the pipes before the bathroom floods.

"Is that a dead rat?" Peter asks as he prodded a hairy glop with the plunger handle.

"No, Bunny, that's my hair," I calmly answer, belying my mixed emotions of panic and depression at the loss of my crowning glory.

Peter tries not to look shocked. I grab the pile and toss it unceremoniously into the trashcan. In most cases hair growth returns to normal once treatment is completed, but the texture and color can be different. *Please, God, anything but pubic hair on my head!*

My hair roots feel and look like porcupine quills and make it especially difficult to put my head on a pillow at night or take my frequent afternoon naps. I feel — and look — like a mangy dog with fleas. This is not my imagination, because Baby tried to groom my head last night. Talk about torture! So after a week of suffering with itchy bald spots and plunging out the drain on a daily basis, I tell Peter, "Let's shave my head. I've had enough slow torture."

I've taken a big step by accepting the fact that although this hair loss will worsen it won't control me.

"Are you sure, Bunny?" Peter asks with one of the saddest looks on his face that I've ever seen. "We could wait a little longer if you want."

"I'm sure. I can't take another moment of this and neither can our drains." I stand in the Jacuzzi and hand him the electric razor and scissors. My hair looks like a nightmare! It's dry and has turned a weird color that defies description other than butt-ugly! We need to put it out of its misery, and mine. I've always said, *to be in pain is human; to suffer is a choice.* I'm choosing not to suffer any longer.

Peter cries silently as he shaves my head. He cries for me because I won't ... I can't. I must be resolute in my decision. This hair is a casualty of war. "This is only temporary and will soon pass," I repeat. My head feels lighter and cold, a strange sensation. As I run my hands over my bald head it feels kind of kinky — as in sexy kinky.

In dream therapy hair is considered thoughts or ideas, so I concentrate on old or negative thoughts and ideas falling to the floor of my mind as my hair falls to the floor of my tub. I've brought a "duality" into the physical realm and hope this spiritual "big medicine" manifests and combines with my conventional medicine to create something greater than the sum of its individual parts. *PMA: positive mental attitude,* I tell myself. *That is what's going to get me through all of this. PMA! If I don't mind the bad stuff, it won't matter.*

When my hair is all shaved off I look like Demi Moore in *G.I. Jane,* kind of feel like her, too. As I look in the mirror and run my hands over my head, I can't get over the contrast of feelings for both my hands and my head. What used to be warm hair is now a cool scalp.

I mentally flash back on the movie and realize that G.I. Jane and I have the same determined look in our eyes as we peer at our new images in the mirror. We can take whatever is thrown at us. We will survive. Did Jane see the people of her inner being stare back at her as I do today? Did her inner warrior grin and say, "Good job." Did her inner psychic smile and say, "This is the beginning of new thoughts and ideas.

 ## Survival Keys

* Embrace your temporal nature. Your body is only temporary, and you are composed of much more than temporary.

* Look to role models. Entertainment heroes can give you strength when your reality is in crisis. Finding inner guidance from strong fictional characters and incorporating them into your inner family can be lifesaving.

* Embrace your inner actor. When life is too difficult to enjoy, fake it till you make it. Pretend to be happy till you are. Be the Xena, Warrior Princess or the GI Jane.

Chapter 15
INTUITION

*Intuition is a spiritual faculty and
does not explain, but simply points the way.*
— Florence Scovel Shinn (1871–1940)

♥ *Affirmation:* I will turn my emotional wounds into
wisdom and use that wisdom for a balanced life.

"When did you become intuitive?" people often ask me.

"I didn't. I was born like this," I reply. "I didn't become, I am, always was."

The first time I heard voices calling my name I was two years of age. It was while my mother held me on her lap and read aloud a book about Peter Cottontail.

"Kathy, what are you looking for?" Mom asked as I twisted and searched the room again.

"Someone's calling my name." "But I can't see them. Where are they?"

"It's just your grandparents telling you from heaven that they love you," she answered and continued to read without giving the voices another thought. This acceptance of the paranormal was pretty astounding for a woman raised by nuns in a Catholic convent, but if Mom was okay with the voices so was I. It wasn't until much later that I found out Mom's parents had been spiritualists who spoke with the dead. Maybe that's why they were so anxious to meet me before they died: takes one to know one.

After Mom's parents came to the U.S. from Germany, Granddad changed their last name from Von Door to his mother's French maiden name. Ashamed of what Germany had done to mankind, he turned his back on his German heritage and embraced the French.

My grandparents were trapeze artists with the Barnum and Bailey Circus and were known as The Flying DeLyons until Grandma fell to her death. Grandpa believed a circus was no place to raise two little girls, so Mom and her younger sister were packed off to a convent in New York with instructions that they could only be adopted together. No one wanted two little girls, so at ages sixteen and seventeen they jumped from the frying pan into the fire and married brothers to escape the nuns.

Later in life I learned that my grandparents had held séances and worked with the Ouija board in their home in Chicago, Illinois. This sounded cool to me, so at fifteen I decided to hold a séance with a Ouija board in Bad Tolz, Germany, where we were stationed. Bad Tolz, now a stronghold of Special Forces, was once the stronghold for Hitler's SS, so it was not unusual for someone to find old guns and other SS treasures beneath the floorboards. Under the base's quadrangle was a catacomb of tunnels the German Army had used to move military equipment and soldiers in the dead of winter. The SS flooded and booby-trapped the tunnels as they fled. This place had many old "spirits," and I wanted to talk to them.

To say the least, this psychic experiment went terribly wrong.

My parents had gone out for dinner, so I invited my friends Steve, Paul, George, and Joann for a Ouija board session. We didn't take it seriously; we just thought we'd have some fun and then study together until my parents came home. We were best friends all through school at Munich American High. We did everything together, and, if it was sneaky, we always got caught. When we skipped school and went to the Munich Zoo, the Baader-Meinhoff terrorist group exploded a car bomb beside a bridge on which we stood.

"Look at that girl on the TV," Mom said and wiped her hands on her apron while watching the evening news in German from the kitchen door. "She looks like Kathy's twin. The young man with her looks like Steve's twin."

My father leaned forward in his chair. "That doesn't *look like* Kathy and Steve, that *is* Kathy and Steve." *Busted!* We were on the evening news!

Having not learned our lesson yet, we set up the Ouija board I'd bought in an antique store. We sat around the living room coffee table on a huge white Flokati sheepskin rug, a memento of an Easter vacation in Greece — and Mom's prize possession.

Giggling and making jokes, we placed our hands on the board and asked if there were any spirits present. Immediately all the lights in the apartment went out. George freaked out, threw his hands up off the board, and hit my twenty-gallon aquarium behind him with his class ring. The tank exploded in the darkness, causing us to scream in unison. The lights came back on just in time for us to witness twenty gallons of water and fish get sucked up by the rug.

"Get a bucket! We have to save my fish!" I cried, gathering as many as I could in my hands. Steve found a bucket under the kitchen sink and we began gingerly peeling fish off the rug. My angelfish's straight feelers had turned curly, like the earlocks of Hasidic Jews. My concern quickly shifted from them to the rug, now doubled in size and weight from twenty gallons of fluid. The apartments below us were in danger of having their ceilings collapse and of us falling through on the rug. I started to hyperventilate.

"We'll drag the rug downstairs to the clothesline in the backyard and hoist it up to drip dry," Steve said to calm me as he tried to lift one of the corners. The rug was heavy, soggy, and almost impossible to move, but we all grabbed a corner, and, using mind over matter, dragged it out the door, down three flights of stairs, and around the building. On the count of three, we hoisted it onto the clothesline, nearly giving ourselves hernias. The clothesline snapped and hit George on the bridge of his nose, right between the eyes. As he let out a howl that could be heard two blocks away in the night, the white rug dropped to the filthy ground.

"What's going on down there?" The commotion had brought the

building's occupants to their back windows. Flashlights shone down on us in the dark. *Busted!*

"Our friend got hit in the nose with the clothesline. Can you take him to the emergency room? We can't drive."

To make a long story short, someone drove George to the hospital for stitches, and with the help of the men in the building, we hung the rug on the clothesline post where it dangled in the dark like a giant, hairy ghost with dirty, shaggy feet.

When my parents returned, Mom immediately asked, "What the hell happened here and where's my rug?"

I answered, "George broke the fish tank, the rug is downstairs drying out, and we're studying." We never told them anything else, but we were busted again!

So ended my first and last séance. I never touched another Ouija board, and I learned an important lesson that night that I still live by today: Never throw your spiritual doors open to everyone in the spirit world and ask them to come in and chat. Chances are very good that they will, and you never know who's wandering around out there or if they'll ever leave. You don't do that with the doors to your home, so don't do it with spiritual doors. "Don't talk to strangers" takes on a whole new level of meaning when it concerns the spirit world. Now, I speak only with people my spirit guides introduce me to — screened friends, not strangers. By the way, no one else's lights went out in the building, though we all shared the same basement fuse box.

Bad Tolz was not the only place that had spirits or ghosts. Berlin was full of them, and they seemed to be attracted to me. They showed up regularly, almost every night, from the witching hour to the hour of souls. They came alone or brought their friends.

I loved living in Berlin, but I hated sleeping there. Culture was everywhere and everything, especially our chic new apartment building, built out of war rubble — pieces, energies, and bodies of the dead. Yeah! After the war, materials were scarce, and everything was recycled without looking at it too closely.

I had four best friends: Deana, Diane, Donna, and Gee-Gee, my invisible friend. Life was good, until I went to sleep. I hated my bedroom. Every night started with the same ritual: close all the closet and dresser drawers, prop open my bedroom door, and make sure the bedroom window was locked. That was phase one. Once in bed, my favorite stuffed animal, Mr. Lion, was on one side of me while my doll Erin was on the other side, against the wall. Gee-Gee was at the foot of the bed. I only had to worry about the head of the bed by the door. I never checked under the bed. What was going to happen tonight would not come from there, and it would be far worse than the boogieman. The boogieman was afraid of my bedroom. Even the cat would rather jump off the third-floor balcony than stay in our apartment at night.

One night was really wild! I awoke to the sound of my closet doors banging open and then soldiers marched down our hallway between the bedrooms. They spoke German and headed toward the far wall at the end of the hallway. They paid little attention to me as they rushed past; however, there was one lone officer, silent except for the sound of his slow boot steps on the hardwood floors and the smell of his cigarette. He stopped at the bedroom door, stared down at me, and smoked. He knew I was there, and I think he knew I knew he was there. He blocked my escape route to my parents' room. On really active nights the windows would blow open, too, and fill my room with cold air. Eventually the officer would walk away. Drenched in perspiration and shivering from fear, I would yell, "Mom, I'm scared!"

"Come on," she would answer. She was used to this. But at least I knew Mom knew that I was heading for her bedroom and if I didn't make it she should come looking for me. I'd grab my pillow and Gee-Gee's hand and run down the hall. Even my imaginary friend was afraid of the ghost officer — and the officer could see Gee-Gee. I'd climb into bed and spoon against Mom's back while Gee-Gee pressed against mine. Mom knew about the cigarette-smoking officer. She didn't hear, smell, or see him, but thank goodness she believed me and let me sleep with her, which I did almost every night for the four years we lived in Berlin.

"Did you wet the bed, Kathy?" she would ask after I climbed in with her. I was so frightened I'd continue to perspire, soaking her sheets, too.

"No, I'm just scared!"

Mom would reach around her body, hug me to her, and we would spoon, just as we had that morning after her death. Forty years later history repeated itself during that tearful hour of souls. Mom's goal at the time of her death was not to frighten me as a spirit, it was to comfort me from beyond and prove that love survives death with the message: You are not alone!

Survival Keys

* Know you have help. Trauma calls to spirits from the other side. They return to the earth plane to give guidance, support, and love to family members and friends in need.

* Connect with guides. Do this through dreams, meditations, and prayer. All are wonderful ways to stay safe during crisis.

Chapter 16

G.I. JANE AND MY NEW BEST FRIENDS — CONSTIPATION AND SWEATS

In the adversity of our best friends we always find something which is not wholly displeasing to us.
— Francois de la Rochefoucauld (1613–1680)

♥ *Affirmation:* Life is a joy filled with delightful surprises.

It's been a week and a day since my first chemotherapy, and I think I'm giving birth to a canoe. I'm so constipated that I call Dr. Barkley on the emergency line.

"I'm so sorry you are in such distress," he sympathized. "Some people experience severe constipation from chemotherapy. Use a warmed Fleet enema. It'll work faster."

So, at ten o'clock at night, I send my poor husband out into the cold to get a Fleet enema from the 24-hour drugstore across town. When he gets home the real fun begins.

"Just stick it in," I yell from my position on my knees clutching my stomach in agony. My intestines have been involuntarily pushing; chemo labor without a spinal block. Peter is more upset than I and paces the floor like an expectant father, enema in hand.

"I'm afraid I'll hurt you, honey. Are you sure you don't want to do this yourself? Is there a special way of putting this in there?" Peter asks as he stands beside me.

"Quickly!" I bark, "Before I'm permanently damaged or explode all over the walls!"

The warm enema works within seconds. I'll now be on a diet of enemas and stool softeners because I never want to go through that again. More shit and giggles, literally.

At midnight, I pull on my yellow ski cap/nightcap — because my head gets so cold — and prepare for sleep. Now I can empathize with bald men, too. I've learned all kinds of lessons and have become so *deep* I can hardly stand myself. What's next?

Tonight's hot flashes and night sweats won't be a problem. After melting in the bed sheets during previous nights, I'm prepared. My three organic cotton T-shirts are on the chair next to the bed. I can grab a bottle of water from the nightstand and drink to extinguish the internal flames, then change into a clean shirt. Hot flashes are different from being hot. This heat is from the inside out, so the best way to deal with it is also from the inside out. Shortly after Hot Flash leaves, his buddy, Night Sweats, makes an appearance. I wake up soaking wet and chilled. The doctor had reassured me that this was a normal side effect of chemo — early menopause. It would pass. But right now I need sleep because tomorrow is a big day. I have my first blood test to see what other, less obvious, side effects I've gotten from all these chemicals. Memories of needles danced in my head like sugarplum fairies. NOT! I settle into bed and count the side effects I've experienced so far on my fingers, starting with "canoe constipation," but before I get very far I fall asleep from another one — fatigue.

"Who is your best IV person?" I ask the admitting nurse the next morning at the Cape Cod Hospital and explain my vein situation. I want the best, and I'm not above being a little pushy about it.

"Let me check some information first." She looked at her computer, then at my arm. "You sound like the poster girl for breast cancer. You're so young, and it doesn't sound like breast cancer runs in your family. I have the perfect IV nurse for you. The emergency room calls for her all the time." I manage a faint smile and sigh with relief.

The admitting nurse shares a wonderful story about a woman who still comes in for her yearly blood tests. She had a seven-centimeter tumor removed eight years ago with eleven lymph nodes involved.

"That was back when chemotherapy wasn't as good as it is today and she's fine. You look like a fighter to me, and I think you'll be fine too." GI Jane nodded.

It is so important to hear these success stories. I need a big dose of hope every day.

Here's another lesson I've learned the hard way. When people start to share a crisis story with me, the first thing I ask is "Does this story have a happy ending? Because if it doesn't, I don't want to hear it!" With a surprised look, they often stop mid-sentence because it doesn't have a happy ending. They don't mean to frighten me; they just want to "share." Unfortunately, unless someone is a crisis survivor they cannot imagine the fear carried by people in therapy. It's much like the fear one carries after a severe car accident. At first it's difficult to even get into a car, let alone hear other people talk about all the people they know who have died in crashes — and the gory details. Over time it's easier to drive a car, and eventually you can even handle stories about accidents — but not while you recover!

I hope someday I'll be strong enough to hear bad stories again, but right now, Life Lesson #7: I only want to hear good stories with happy endings, and I'm not afraid to say so! The story my tennis friend told me of the woman dying in the emergency room from vomiting with a tube down her throat is the last scary story I care to hear during treatment. If there's another important story that needs to be told to save my life — *tell it to Peter!*

Within five minutes a stout, elderly lady with curly gray hair and a lovely smile shows up and introduces herself as the IV nurse. "Oh, there's a good one right here," she says, peering closely at my arm, and she hasn't even applied the tourniquet yet. Her confidence is infectious. "I'm going to use a baby needle so it won't hurt you. It may take a little longer to fill the tube, but it won't cause your vein to blow up." I tell her I have no plans for the rest of the day. "Would you please write down your name and the days you work?" If I had to get down on my knees and beg, I would. She smiles and hands me her card.

"Ask for me anytime," she says, taping gauze over the puncture. "I'll be here."

I've never had such an easy blood test in my life. This woman must be an angel. She's *my* angel now and I have her name and number.

After that wonderful story about the woman who had cancer so long ago with so many lymph nodes involved, I decide that I need more good stories, so I bought a book from the bookstore, an anthology of cancer survivors sharing stories and giving advice. Each page has a paragraph that gives their accounts and thoughts on what to expect during treatment. It's a good thing I've been reading it in my bubble bath with scented candles and soft music because I'm reduced to a puddle of tears. I've never read anything so scary or depressing. *The Texas Chainsaw Massacre* wasn't this bad. I refused to read any more of the book and threw it in the trash once I found it through my tears. I need something written with a sense of humor because crisis is depressing enough. Irving S. Cobb stated it perfectly: "Humor is merely tragedy standing on its head with its pants torn."

I already know there are side effects and problems with treatment. I'm living them. Give me hope and solutions. Is that possible, or am I shooting for the moon? Medical books are too difficult for my chemo brain to understand, and other books don't deal with the psychic, spiritual, dream, or nightmare aspects of illness. I'm sure I'm not the first person to have nightmares during trauma, and I'm sure I won't be the last. So far, the information I've used the most is my personal experience caring for a dying mother. Who would have thought I'd need that to save myself?

I lean back, remove the washcloth covering my eyes, and gaze up at the full moon. I'm relieved to see my old friend looking down on me. The man in the moon and I are so emotionally connected now. He's always there during the worst of times, shining a pure light on difficult situations. That light is like God's flashlight at the end of the long tunnel of life. It illuminates the way when I feel lost, which is so often. Finding myself is challenging.

I've changed. This confuses me because I respond to life's situations differently now: Situations that I once tolerated, I no longer accept. I'm emotional about things that would have had little effect on me in the past. I'm evolving and don't recognize myself when I look in the mirror. But I like this new me. I put my hands on my face and remember the words of Lewis Carroll, author of *Alice in Wonderland*: "Who in the world am I? Ah, that's the great puzzle."

It's more than physical changes like hair loss and weight loss and dark circles beneath bloodshot eyes. It is an emotional and mental change. I'm morphing into a different person moving in a different direction, and I've decided not to try to control it but rather see where it takes me. Relinquishing control is a new and somewhat scary concept that is also exciting, because I wake up as a different person every morning and don't know where or when the changes will end. Does the caterpillar know what it will look like when it emerges from the cocoon? I had similar feelings when I began college. Maybe I'm graduating from UHK — the University of Hard Knocks. Is this yet another silver lining? Sometimes we must create our silver linings. I'm going to dry my eyes and prepare for my second chemo treatment, right now, in the tub, gazing at my friend Mr. Moon. My next treatment is coming so soon that it seems like hours, rather than days, away.

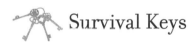 Survival Keys

* Grow through Trauma. Trauma is an important time of growth.

* Learn from new experiences. We develop depth of character that would not be possible without the baptism by fire crisis gives us.

* Prepare to be enlightened. People in crisis often experience spiritual enlightenment. Perhaps it is God's finger tapping our shoulder as a reminder.

Chapter 17
MOVING FORWARD

It is not the mountain we conquer but ourselves.
— Sir Edmund Hillary (1919–2008)

♥ *Affirmation:* I will face my problems one at a time,
even when they refuse to get in line.

We left for the Dana-Farber Institute on another cold rainy Tuesday morning. Poor Peter had to stop twice at bathrooms along the way. I'm not sure if it's due to anxiety or the warm water I drank. I know he dreads my pathetic whine: "Bunny, I have to pee." Next time, I'll take a thermos full of hot tea and drink it thirty minutes from the hospital. These potty stops have made us late again, which causes a domino effect of delays, but this time I'm able to get the front desk with my special phone number.

The nurse drawing blood stuck me only once; then I was sent to Deana for my next needle. As she searches my arm, I tell her about my IV angel on Cape Cod.

"That's great, but you tell her this vein right here is mine. And that goes for the blood test nurses here, too," she says pointing to the large vein that runs down the under-side of my forearm. After soaking my arm in hot water, I return it to her pink, warm, and wrapped in a towel. She leads me to my quiet room. Peter had brought along a meditation CD from Cindy. No sooner had I begun listening than the pain therapist arrives and soothes me further with her lovely conversation. All this leads to a successful one-try-only needle insertion. I'm so relieved I almost cry. With the blood test done and the chemo needle in place,

I'm ready to get this party on the road as soon as the blood-test results come in. Dr. Barkley always tests his patients to be sure blood levels have returned to an acceptable level for chemo. *Whatever ... Just do me and get me outta here!*

"No chemo for you today," Dr. Barkley says as he wheels himself over to where I sit. "Your test shows your blood levels are still too low for treatment. Sorry. Let's see how they are in three days. Go home, rest, and get another blood test on Saturday. I think you'll be able to take your treatment on Monday."

"Is this normal?" I ask. I have to go through this again in five days with another blood test in-between. The more I think about it the more upset I become.

"Not all blood levels recover when we expect," he replies. "Some people take extra days to recuperate, and yes, it's normal for those people. Your levels seem to be dropping later and recovering later as well. To save you this inconvenience again, take a blood test at the Cape two days before you come in to see if you need extra recovery time." Life Lesson #4: "There are no norms, only you," seems to apply to every aspect of life.

As cute as Dr. Barkley looks on that stool with his bowtie and vest, I want to grab him by his tiny throat and yell, "Do you know what I had to go through to prepare myself for this treatment? Give it to me anyhow!" But I behave myself and let the nurse remove my IV.

Driving home, I fluctuate between relief and depression — relief at not going through all that chemo shit, but depressed because of two extra blood tests including more chemo shit in five days. Oh, well, I'll worry about that later. Right now, I need a bathroom ... again!

Two days later my levels had recovered and the results were faxed to Dr. Barkley.

As soon as we get off the elevator, I make a beeline to the nearest sink and soak my arm in hot water. *Bad move!* Warm water works in many ways, and I'm about to wet my pants. I grab a towel for my arm, or to use on the floor if I don't make it to the bathroom, and run for the toilet, praying it's empty. I feel like I'm losing my mind from my toilet fixation. This constant peeing can't be normal. Is that tiny light in the tunnel another train coming at me?

"That is a normal side effect of chemotherapy," Dr. Barkley reassures me from his little stool. "You need to continue to drink lots of fluids to clear your system, so look for a bathroom before you really need it. Since you'll use the bathroom throughout the night, some spouses find the sleep disturbance difficult and move into another bedroom for the duration of treatment."

Once again, my pretreatment blood test didn't go smoothly and my nurse and pain specialist, called in by Maureen, the head nurse, welcome me back to my quiet room. Guess I still don't play well with others. How depressing. As I settle into my chair, Peter puts earphones on my head and turns up my classical music. The Ativan I took earlier takes effect, and I feel good as Deana glides the second needle into my vein on the first try. I'm almost halfway through with chemotherapy. It hasn't been as bad as I imagined, because the hospital staff is so kind. In a few hours, I'll be over the hump and down the other side of chemo's bumpy road.

"Two down, two to go," I whisper.

"What did you say?" Peter asks, pulling the earphone off one of my ears. "We must celebrate with a nice dinner downtown." I imagine food in front of me and almost puke.

"Yeah." I turn my head so he won't see my eyes fill with tears. Is it the nausea, the chemo, my physical weakness, or memories of a previous life? I'm not sure — none or all of the above. Snow begins to fall outside the window. It looks so pure and serene.

To my surprise, Deana says she needs my coveted "quiet room" for another patient, and without giving me time to react to this change in my program, escorts me into the infusion room and sits me in a reclining chair. I've just been pushed onto the playground with the rest of the kids. Will we like each other? Patients waved as I walked past them. There are no strangers here. I feel accepted. Hmm, did the nurse really need that room, or did she wean me away from my isolation? These nurses are so smart!

The infusion room takes on a surreal atmosphere as I watch women glide by, led by hospital personnel in white gowns. It reminds me of the dream I had called The Room Between Realms. This time, instead of being led past groups of stationary women, I watch them being led past me in this infusion room between realms. Is life mimicking my dream, or was my dream mimicking life — art mimicking life mimicking art? Which is reality and which is the nightmare, and will I ever wake up?

My attention is drawn to the flutter of black robes. Seated across from me in an infusion chair is a Muslim woman in a full traditional burka, complete with string between the eyes and long black gloves. Only her eyes are not hidden — and one arm, which is hooked up to IV bags and is being lovingly stroked by her husband seated beside her. I watch her study me. The ravages of chemotherapy are hidden beneath her black burka, mine beneath my blond wig. Although we have different cultures, beliefs, and clothing, cancer has united us in the struggle to live. Cancer truly is an equal-opportunity disease that creates universal suffering. All you have to do to get it is be alive.

I was taught that it's bad manners to stare, but I cannot tear my eyes from this woman. Although her body is hidden, she exudes dignity. She murmurs something to her husband who glances over at me just as Peter takes my hand and kisses it. With that kiss, I realize that my burka'd friend and I have something else in common — love. Obviously, Muslim families love their women, too. The Muslim man caressing his wife's bare arm loves her as much as my Christian husband kissing my hand loves me. I smile at them and then shift my gaze to the window to give them privacy in this public place.

While I wait for the green light to proceed with my treatment, I reflect on just how much my life has changed since my birthday, just three months ago. My old obsessions used to be tennis, shopping, and partying with my old friends. My new obsessions are veins, nausea, and bathrooms with my new friends — stool softeners and Fleet enemas. Yes, I've come a very long way. Will I ever get back there? Have I changed too much to ever find my way, or want to?

"This is Doreen, the floor superintendent. She organizes everything here," Deana says as Doreen extends her hand and shakes mine.

"I remember you from a few weeks ago," Doreen says with a grin. Suddenly I remember her too. I think I told her to go get me a Chinese anesthesiologist from the basement of Brigham and Women's Hospital and she may have been the person who called the psychiatrist. I feel embarrassed, but she's so friendly that my awkwardness disappears. Doreen strikes me as an extremely advantageous person to know.

I put my feet up, wait for the blood test to green light my therapy, and peek at the other patients reclined in their chairs. Most of them are peeking back at me. We don't want to be so bold as to gawk at each other. Everyone, including the people with bandages around their bruised faces from surgery, has a sense of dignity. There is a good feeling here. Many women wear attractive hats or have wrapped beautiful scarves around their heads. I was very impressed that Doreen recognized me with my wig on, because this is the first time I've worn it. These nurses seem to be aware of everything and they don't miss a beat.

Doreen reappears with another patient. Speaking to the other girl about me, she says, "Look at her. She looks great, she's glowing." I wonder if Doreen is pulling my leg, but Deana and Peter both say I look really good today. Make-up is magic.

I've got the go-ahead for my chemo. It's a good thing, because they've already filled me up with everything except a keg of beer for hydration. While Deana monitors my purple Kool-Aid chemo she asks, "What perfume are you wearing? You smell so good." "Calyx by Prescriptive," I answer. (At least this time it wasn't surgical scrub soap.) Calyx is one of the few pure fragrances that can erase that rancid oil smell from my pores after treatment.

As woozy as I feel, I tell Peter we should celebrate our success. I say "our" because when things go badly for me, they go badly for him, and when they go well for me, oh, happy days! We'll have a romantic dinner in downtown Boston, during a raging snowstorm made romantic by firelight and love.

Survival Keys

✳ Celebrate. Celebrating milestones, no matter how small, is important when moving through the dark tunnel of crisis.

✳ Create. We have the ability to manifest, so create a little heaven along the way.

✳ Don't stop; keep moving forward. Life is movement. In the words of Winston Churchill, "If you're going through hell, keep going."

Chapter 18

VISUALIZATION, MEDITATION, AND "THEM"

*Nothing would be more tiresome than eating and drinking
if God had not made them a pleasure as well as a necessity.*
— Voltaire (1694–1778)

♥ *Affirmation:* Loving myself heals my life. I nourish my mind,
body, and soul with dreams and meditation.

Peter wraps his scarf around me twice, props me gently against a quaint gas lamppost, like those that line the streets of downtown Boston, and says, "Stay right here. I'll see if the restaurant is open." Like I had the energy to go anywhere. He had realized within minutes of our walk that I was too weak to make it to the restaurant and back if it were closed.

At least he didn't tie me to the lamppost. People on cell phones try to dig their cars out of three feet of snow while I don't have the strength to brush the flakes off my nose or eyelashes as they melt and slide down my face. One man with bright red gloveless hands and wearing only a sweater pushes snow off his car. He's probably some poor schmuck transferred from California whose closest experience to a snowstorm is a snow cone.

I feel compelled to warn him about yellow snow but don't have the energy for conversation. I'll need it if the snowplow comes by and covers me before Peter gets back. It's happened before to children and to pets tied to posts. I'll have to bark like a dog and hope someone hears and digs me out. It's already dark at four o'clock. The orange light from gas lamps shimmers on falling snow. The street looks like a Kinkade painting. As ripples of light play off the shadows, waves of nausea wash over me.

True to his word, Peter reappears, a devilish grin on his face. "You'll love this restaurant. It's the perfect, romantic place you wanted."

It's a lovely little spot in the basement of an old building made cozy by brick walls warmed by the light of tiny votive candles on red-and-white-checkered tablecloths. Delicious aromas precede plates of steaming food. I didn't eat much, but what I ate was well worth the hiccups.

We celebrated my halfway point with a shared glass of red wine. Drinking one by myself would have knocked me on the floor. (I should do that before my next blood test. Couldn't hurt.)

Later, at home, my guides join the celebration by giving me my color and number.

Every morning and evening, and often at naptime, I do a visualization and meditation. I started this even before I played the meditation tape Cindy gave me, surprisingly similar to my own meditation. My guides led me through my first meditation. The colors they gave me to visualize with each chakra and its location were different from anything in books. Maybe this deviation from the norm was just for me because I'm not in the norm of life — I'm in a fight to the death.

My meditation place is a temple high in the sky of my mind. It overlooks the ocean on one side and a rainforest on the other. It's a beautiful place filled with sounds of life. Clouds act as pathways traveled by spiritual guides. In my meditation, I ask God to send his healing golden light of health and love into the crown of my head and down into my chakras where it is caught in crystal chalices. I stand in light that surrounds me like a waterfall. I feel my seventh, violet, chakra of higher spirit fill with warm liquid light, which overflows into my sixth, blue, charka, located between my eyes, that stores the psychic gifts I use to access my spirit guides. Warmth fills my sixth chakra and overflows into my fifth, purple, throat chakra, used for communication, until that chalice overflows into the fourth, green and pink, chakra of my breasts, love and relationships.

I thank God for filling this fourth chalice. It fills both breasts before flowing into my hands. Any negativity is washed out of my fingertips and thrown into the purple flame of Saint Germain where it is converted into positive energy and returned to the universe. Next, the golden liquid flows into my stomach, abdomen, pancreas, gall bladder, liver, spleen, kidneys, ovaries, uterus, and bladder, then washes through my third, red, chakra of forgiveness. Forgiveness is freedom from the past. Again, the purple flame of Saint Germain cleanses any negativity. Warm light flows down my legs to my knees and into my second, orange, chakra. I claim this as my personal chakra because I was given the number two with the color orange in my color and number dream. I visualize all the people who constitute my inner self being washed with this healing light. As it washes down my legs to my first, yellow, chakra, my tribe chakra, the light connects all my tribes, both here on the earth plane and on the other side of life — the dead. Finally, the golden light flows out through the bottoms of my feet and connects me to the earth. The warmth makes me break out in perspiration. Next, an angel appears with a tuning fork, hits the fork on her hand to create a perfect tone, and passes it over me. As I become one with the sound my body vibrates in this harmonious perfection of tone.

I've used this meditation since I began treatment, but tonight something interesting happens: As I complete the meditation, a voice in my mind says, "*Wait.*" All the crystal chalices combine to become one, brilliant with all the colors of my chakras, like a giant diamond, and it fills with golden liquid. "Drink in the name of the Father, Son, and Holy Spirit."

Okay, I think, and drink the warm liquid with my mind. *Is that all?*

"*Lift up a portion of the skin on your arm and look under it.*"

I mentally lift a flap of skin and see bright golden light. Another voice says, "*She's really cookin' now!*"

Is that all? I ask the voices again.

"*Wait.*" Two angels appear on either side of me and brush off my aura with fans made of three large white feathers. Next, my spirit guides give me symbols to go with each chakra. They are different from anything I've seen in books.

Am I done, now? I ask the voice a third time.

"Sleep," the voice answers gently, and a hand extends from time and space to give me a beautiful yellow dandelion. *"This is your flower. Use it as a wand to touch anything you wish to change. Keep it safe in your heart chakra and it will be there whenever you need it."*

After falling asleep, I hear the song *Tiny Bubbles,* by Hawaiian singer Don Ho, playing in my mind. I'm on a sunny beach making red and white bubbles by dancing in the surf with a bubble kit. Bubbles transform into transparent chakra colors and absorb into my body through my skin, nose, and ears. I realize I'm asleep and having a lucid dream.

I believe the bubbles in my dream were my blood cells healing. Ocean is the Christ symbol. An ocean full of Christ washed and healed my cells. This was a lucid healing dream. Dandelion means tooth of the lion because of the outline of the leaves. It is also an edible weed said to have health benefits.

"Ask and you shall receive." This is a powerful reminder of how the spirit within us is capable of manifesting those things in life that are important to us, including overcoming trauma, crisis, and illness.

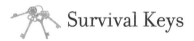 Survival Keys

* Choose your words wisely. We might not always get what we ask for in life, but we will get what we need, so choose your words wisely because the universe is always listening.

Chapter 19
VISITING SPIRITS

If we are facing in the right direction,
All we have to do is keep on walking.
— Buddhist proverb

♥ *Affirmation:* I choose to love everyone to the best of my ability.

I have a new friend. A couple of months ago I met a lovely woman named Patricia Rook who helped Peter with his book, *Pope Annalisa*. Patricia is an internationally published English author who doesn't drive and teaches college. Peter described her as a Miss Marple teacher type who demands the very best from her students.

As we drive to her house to pick up his manuscript, he mentions that Patricia has a son who recovered from pancreatic cancer and that Patricia has written books on hauntings around the world. My antenna went up. What would she think of me? Would she "feel" my intuitive vibrations and refuse to work on Peter's book, much like my frightened housekeeper who quit?

As it turned out, I knew the moment I met Patricia that I had known her in a previous life. She was part of my tribe. We became instant friends when she gave me a big motherly hug.

"I don't think Patricia is usually that friendly to strangers. I'm surprised she took to you so quickly," Peter said in the car on the way home.

"I'm so cute with my little bald head. How could anyone resist me?" I joked.

Well, today Patricia phones me with a request I hope I can fill. She asks me to meditate on her son to see what information I get on his health, so I do a meditation and refer to the person as "Patricia's son." From a guide, I receive the information that her son has a peptic ulcer.

"Oh," she replied. "That's my other son. I already know that. I meant my son Tom."

Well, that's interesting. I didn't know she had two sons.

I've never done this before, but Patricia wants me to contact Tom's guides to see if they'll be with him during his intestinal exploratory surgery at 5:30 a.m. tomorrow. She's worried about his heart from all the chemotherapy he's taken over the years for his cancer. He is one of two people in the world to survive pancreatic cancer that spread to his liver and bones. Tom has not been able keep food down and is on a feeding tube.

Patricia and I have discussed some of the things Peter and I have done, especially communication with spirit guides. The problem is that contacting and talking to my guides has always been on their terms. They pop up and summon me. I've never actually summoned them until just now, with her other son. I really do want to help. I just hope I can. Whenever I wonder what to do and how to begin, my ego gets in the way with limiting thoughts. *What if you can't help? Patricia might think you're just a head case to be carted off to the nearest funny farm. She is helping Peter with his book. If I can't help I'll still have to face her again and that might be really embarrassing. This is not some stranger whom I'll never have contact with again; this is a friend!*

"I'll see what I can do," I promise Patricia over the phone. "I've never done this before, but let's see what happens when I try to contact Tom's guides." I can tell she's very worried about him, but she thanks me with her lovely British accent and says, "Whatever you can do, dear, will be greatly appreciated."

As soon as I hang up, I say a little prayer and explain the situation to God and any guides who might be listening. I want them to know that I'm very unsure of myself.

"Ask and you shall receive," a voice whispered. Was that me or a guide? *"Stop thinking so much. Open your mind, trust in yourself and believe."* Then the voice was gone.

At 4:43 the next morning, I awoke from a sound sleep and looked at the alarm clock. This is unusual for me because I don't wake up before 10:00 a.m., and on chemotherapy I might sleep until 11:00 or longer, sometimes all day.

It's fifteen minutes until Tom's surgery, and I didn't have any pop-up dreams or information — nothing at all. This isn't good, I thought. I decided to meditate and try to have a pop-up dream about Tom. I call on my and Tom's guides and thank them for whatever help they could give. No sooner have I begun to meditate and ask whether any of Tom's spiritual guides or angels are here, than I feel pulled out of my bedroom and see with my inner eyes, for lack of a better term, that I'm in a hospital room with a man attached to tubes and IVs. I hope this is Tom, because I've never seen a photo or had any contact with him.

"Is a guide here for Tom?" I ask, looking around the room, rather shocked to be there. If this is not Tom's room, will someone tell me to leave?

A soft female voice echoes in reply: "I'm here. My name is Portia."

I scan the room but see no one except the man in the hospital bed.

"Portia, are you going to stay with Tom throughout his surgery?"

"Yes. I'll be here."

Good! I think. Just as I thank Portia for staying with Tom and for speaking with me, I'm pulled out of the hospital room and back into my bed while trying to remember Portia's name. *Remember the sports car.* When I meditate again at 6:30 and 7:30, I ask Portia if she is still with Tom. A voice gently answers, "Yes." This time, however, I didn't astral travel to the hospital room. Her voice just came to me across time and space.

"Hello, Patricia? I have some information and a name for you," and I tell her everything that had happened. "Does the name Portia ring a bell? She might be someone who died and is not a guide, because I couldn't see her. I could only hear her."

"No, dear. I know all the names in my family tree because of my genealogy studies, and that name is unfamiliar to me. But thank you for trying."

Patricia has an advanced degree in archaeology and anthropology from Oxford University and does genealogy as a hobby between writing murder mysteries.

Well, so much for that, I think as I pad around the kitchen in slippers and bathrobe. *I gave it my best shot, but this is not one of my gifts.* I sit on our patio, sip coffee, watch the tide recede over the grass flats, and say a prayer for Tom, who's still in surgery.

Two days later the phone rings. It's Patricia. "I've just spoken to Tom and have something to share with you that is quite amazing. You were in Tom's room. I told him about Portia and he became quite emotional. It seems that when he was in military intelligence he worked closely with a woman named Portia in Israeli intelligence. She was killed, and Tom avenged her death. He never told anyone because it was classified information, which also upset him. Even though Portia was murdered many years ago, he remembers her fondly. So you see, dear, you were right on the mark. Portia is not a guide; she's a dead friend."

I was flabbergasted. Did I really astral travel? Did I really hear Portia? Why did I see Tom but not her? These psychic experiences never ceased to amaze me and often left me with more questions than answers, but I realized then that I had just been blessed with a new gift, maybe two. Portia would not be the only friend of Tom's I would meet from the other side. Throughout his surgeries during my treatments, there would be more meetings, including one with his other Israeli partner, David, who was also killed by Palestinians.

A few days later, Tom had complications from his surgery, and again Patricia asked me to check on him. This time, when I astral traveled to a position beside Tom's bed, David was there, wearing a brown leather bomber jacket. He turned to face me with a smile and introduced himself. David was with Portia, whom, again, I could only hear. When I relayed this to Tom, he immediately recognized David's name and description, including the jacket his old friend had always worn.

It was after this second surgery that I found out why I couldn't see Portia: She had been blown up by the Palestinians. This was her way of confirming her presence. When people pass over in a certain way, perhaps from a heart attack, they will often appear with a glow-ing heart so that there is immediate recognition and validation. "*Oh, yes, he died of a heart attack.*" I don't know why I was so surprised by all this; after all, I had been hearing the dead since I was two and see-ing them since second grade in Berlin. In childhood I had Gee-Gee, my imaginary friend, to keep me out of trouble with spirits. Now I had spirit guides who took me to trouble and spirits. Why didn't my guides protect me as a little girl from that German officer ghost who terrorized me in the middle of the night?

When I think of Gee-Gee now, I think of the biblical verse "When I was a child, I spoke as a child, I understood as a child, I thought as a child …" (1 Corinthians 13:11). Is Gee-Gee now a guide who inter-acts with me as an adult?

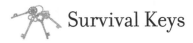 Survival Keys

* Validate. Spirits who share names that can be validated in life prove that there is life after death.

* Focus. Facts can be stranger than fiction, but in Cancerland, which is which? The key is to focus on what is right for you.

Chapter 20

MEDIA OVERLOAD DURING TREATMENT

Cancer — the equal-opportunity disease
no one should have the opportunity to have!
— Kathleen O'Keefe-Kanavos

♥ *Affirmation:* I am at peace with my correct choices.

October, which is Breast Cancer Awareness Month, is seven months away, yet I'm watching marches and telethons on TV now. The Cancer Society does a great job of educating the mainstream population on breast cancer, but right now I'm overly aware of it. These programs scare the daylights out of me, but it's my responsibility to shield myself from this overload, even when it graces my TV again in October. "Boo! You have cancer! Trick or Treat! Stop the world, I wanna get off!" I've cried so hard that my ears itch and I can no longer see the TV screen, so I turn it off and sit in silence. But I can't turn off my tears. Crying and being scared can't be good for me now. I need to be happy and positive. This is no time for me to watch *The Life and Death of Linda McCartney*, which mirrors *Love Story*, the 1970 film starring Ali MacGraw and Ryan O'Neal.

I pray that someday when I'm healthy again I can give back to society, too, like those brave women marching with only one or no breasts and their supportive families. If Linda, with all the money, power, support, and undying love of her husband couldn't beat this miserable disease, what in the world makes me think I can? While the majority of the

117

population is limited as to treatment choices and hospitals, Linda could go anywhere in the world to find the best hospitals and doctors. As a matter of fact, she did, but it didn't help her. She still died, leaving behind a grieving husband and family. I know Peter would hold my hand to the very end, too, but I don't want this life to end yet. Could the pain on his face at the moment of my death hold me here past my time? I hope so!

I think I should stop writing, because all of these dire memories are sending my inner children screaming through the halls of my mind yelling, "We're all gonna die!" as my inner adults try to catch them. *Find something humorous on TV and get out of this black funk.* I flip through the channels as fast as I can to avoid any more sad stuff and settle on a comedy with The Three Stooges. Yes, this will do just fine. I feel better already. Finally all is quiet in my inner halls as the children settle down to watch TV, too.

So much for a quiet body and mind. Yesterday my blood pressure was so high the doctors sent me to an ophthalmologist in Boston for a complete eye exam. They're concerned that the elevated pressure could affect my vision. (That's not what I need to hear to bring it down!) Actually, I've heard my heart beating in my ears for the past two months. The cousin who sent me the information on Dr. Nagourney drove me to my ophthalmologist appointment.

"Oh, my! Let's try that again. That can't be right," the technician said and peered at the instrument that blows a puff of air to check eye pressure. My eyes really dislike that test and have a way of shutting themselves at the exact moment the air is expelled. I couldn't time it better if I tried a hundred times. Maybe my eye is psychic. After the second try, she gives me a funny look and says, "Please sit in the hall. I'll get the doctor."

My ears are ringing, and I can hear the blood rushing in them. *Shhh,* I say to myself. *Shhh.* Slowly the swishing and ringing diminish.

"My name is Doctor Chann. I understand you're going through chemotherapy," the tall, slender Asian woman said, extending a delicate hand. "Since the pressure in your eyes is so high, I'll dilate the pupils and check the cornea. Can someone drive you home?

The yellow drops sting and make me sneeze. "That happens all the time," she says, mistaking my look of horror for embarrassment. I'm afraid I've blown all the liquid out my nose from my eye and she'll need to add more drops.

"Blood pressure can rise during treatments or traumas, but it's often temporary."

I feel that I'm in good hands, and wipe my nose again as I nod my head in agreement.

After thirty minutes of lights and drops, Dr. Chann announces that she doesn't think I need drops to reduce the pressure because it's not as high as she had previously suspected. "I'd like to see you in a month," she says and walks me to the door. It's a good thing she does, because my depth perception is off from the drops. I keep missing the door handle as I try to close it behind me.

I couldn't help but wonder if saying "Shhh" had brought down my blood pressure and the pressure in my eyes, because the first technician with the puffs of air certainly looked concerned. From now on every time I hear my blood pressure in my ears, I'll sit quietly, calm myself, and say, shhh, shhh. I can do it. I just did, so I can do it again in the face of any crisis.

Baby Cakes, my cat, has been a great help with my meditations. He seems to understand that I'm not well and has been trying, in his own special way, to care for me. Baby has always been exceptional, but now he's showing a side of himself that we've never seen before. He's a furry little healer armed with a vicious healing purr.

Baby Cakes was our Easter-Bunny kitten with his white body and pink nose and ears: the points of a flame point Birman. Born in October (breast cancer month), he sprang into our lives in April and has been with us for fourteen years. Little did I know the day I snatched him, sick, sneezing, and coughing, from a cage in a mall pet shop, that years later he would be my lucky charm with his four white rabbit feet, intelligent blue eyes, and a language of tweets, chirps, and barks. He's my tiny white knight in furry armor who guards me during naptime and sits on my feet in the bathroom to keep them warm during my nightly toilet runs.

The chemotherapy has caused ringing in my ears to the point of distraction, especially when I lie down for a nap or at night when I try to sleep. So, Baby climbs up on the bed with me, wraps his paws around my neck, places his head on mine, and purrs as loudly as he can into my ear. While I meditate on returning my body (and his) to perfection, I hear Baby repeat in my ear, *"Puuurrrr-fect. Puuuurrr-fect."* I never remember falling asleep. I just know that when I awaken, Baby is still in the same position, standing guard over me and continuing his softer, quieter healing mantra *"Puuurrr-fect. Puuurrr-fect."*

 ## Survival Keys

* Don't mind it, and it won't matter. If you don't mind it (take "it" into your consciousness) it won't "matter" (become matter or manifest physically and take on form to become gray matter in your brain: intelligence).

* Pay attention to pets. Tune in to the companionship loyal pets are always ready to provide.

Chapter 21
THE IDES OF MARCH

The adventure of life is to learn. The purpose of life is to grow.
The nature of life is to change. The challenge of life is to care.
The opportunity of life is to serve. The secret of life is to dare.
The spice of life is to befriend. The beauty of life is to give.

The joy of life is to Love.
— William Arthur Ward (1921–1994)

♥ *Affirmation:* Today I will dare to continue to grow.

"Beware the Ides of March," the soothsayer warned Julius Caesar. He might as well be warning me. Throughout history March 15 came to represent a day that set off a ripple of repercussions in one's life. Some things never change. Rather than a knife in the back, like Caesar, I just got one in the heart.

My peaceful nap with Baby Cakes is interrupted by an unexpected phone call that quickly turns to dread. I had been avoiding telling Dad about my cancer, and life just solved that problem for me.

"I'd love to come and help you recover from surgery, but I don't think my doctors will release me," began my phone call from hell to my shocked father. I'm almost halfway through my chemo and thought I could complete it without worrying him, but things don't always work out as planned. When you ask the universe to help you solve your problems, it does.

Dad needs a double hernia operation. He hoped I would go down to Florida to help him with his recovery. And I would if I could — but

121

I can't. Now I've added a big headache to his abdominal pain. To comfort me, and act as if he understands my every word, Baby sits on my lap and studies my face. He reacts to each expression change while kneading my leg for emotional support during one of the most difficult conversations I've ever had, telling Dad, who lost his wife of fifty years to colon cancer, that his daughter is now fighting for her life with breast cancer. The cat is out of the bag.

"Are you going to be okay, babe?" he asks with a slight tremble to his voice that exposed his fear for me.

"I'm going to be fine, Daddy. I'm almost through my treatment," I white lied.

"There are so many new treatments out now, compared to when your mother went through this. They have treatments now where they take your own blood and make chemotherapy out of it. So don't be afraid. You're going to be okay. I'll go and stay with Tommy after my surgery, and he'll take good care of me. You just worry about your-self right now."

"I will, Dad, so don't worry about me. This is just another small bump in the road of life."

"That's the attitude! Love you, babe."

"I love you, too, Daddy."

As I hang up I get a flash of my father crying and know it was prob-ably his guides talking to my guides talking to me. I call my brother and asked him to call Dad and reassure him. Tommy didn't know anything about Dad's upcoming operation. Dad hadn't told him, just as I hadn't told Dad. How the universe works is absolutely amazing. Now everyone knows!

Dad is a very private person. I'll bet I get this habit of sharing as little information as possible from him. It's probably genetic. Peter always asks me to tell him what's bothering me. He has even tried to teach me to complain and whine, to no avail. Dad is happiest when dropped alone out of a plane in some remote area with just a knife and compass. As a Green Beret, he lived with the Montagnards in Vietnam and headed search-and-destroy missions in the jungle with-out a base camp of his own. He never talked or complained about the war. The war was what it was. He made the most of it and moved on. Mom and I would have known little of what he did in Vietnam had not one of the injured soldiers appeared on our doorstep in Fayetteville, North Carolina, home of the Green Berets. Over lunch, he told us his story of being rescue by Dad. Jack had been buried alive by his buddy after they were ambushed by the Vietcong and shot, he in the left lung and foot and his buddy in the hip and shoulder. Jack's buddy buried him under a pile of jungle debris in the hope that the Vietcong would pass over him and continue their chase. In the meantime, the pursued soldier ran into Dad's search-and destroy-party, which had been apprised of the firefight by local farmers. The buddy led Dad to Jack, whose collapsed lung had caused him to pass out, which in turn saved his life because the Vietcong couldn't hear him breathing beneath the debris as they stood above him. Imagine being so close to death it actually saves your life.

Dad never spoke of these war stories and made the transition back to "normal life" relatively well, though he slept in a separate bedroom, and we had to call to him from the doorway before entering. His reactions were still lightning fast and in automatic-reflex mode — and that made him dangerous. Even though the conscious mind may be able to perceive and adapt to a different time and space such as "later and safely back home," the subconscious mind is always in a state of *now*. It melds the past, present, and future while focusing on survival.

I wonder how long it will be before I return to normal life. How long before my subconscious, which now perceives danger at every turn, readjusts to life after this is all over. Hmmm. What if this is never all over? I don't want to go there. Time enough for thoughts like that later if things take a turn for the worse. Can they get worse than this phone call? *"Oh, yes,"* a voice says. *Shut up!* I answer. *That was a rhetorical question.* Back to Dad:

Now I have to worry about him worrying about me while I worry about him. "Could things get any more complicated?" I ask Baby Cakes as I stroke him. He answers with a tweeter. Just the simple act of petting him has a calming effect on me. I don't feel quite as anxious. No wonder they take pets to visit people in retirement homes.

"Come on, Baby, I need another naptime puurr session. That call knocked the wind out of my sails. What do you think of that idea?" I asked the tiny white face with beseeching blue eyes. *"Puuuurrr-fect,"* he replies and jumps down to lead the way to the bedroom.

My phone call from Dad was followed by an interesting dream last night that involved Billy, the developmentally disabled teenager.

Peter and I are in northern Florida. It starts to snow so we drive to southern Florida's beautiful sunny beaches. Happily, I ride my bike to a café on stilts on the beach. People gather outside a large picture window. Billy comes up to me and says, "Why is your head like that?" I realize that I'm not wearing my wig, and I'm shocked that no one else noticed. I turned to the boy and demand, "How can you ask me that and make me feel bad?" I'm annoyed with him for making me self-conscious when I was having a good time.

A man about thirty years old steps over from the group, puts his arm around the boy, and says, "Remember, we went through this, too. We decided, too, remember?"

"Oh, yeah," the boy answers as he's led over to the window to look out at the ocean with all the other people.

Interpretation: This dream is about psychological problem solving and inner unification. In it I become balanced, centered in self, and one with God. I am challenged by my less-developed but true self only to find that all of my selves have agreed to go through this crisis with me. I'm not alone. This is a dream of integration, balance, and protection that reinforces the concept: to effectively battle illness we must get in touch with all our inner selves and work together toward the goal of survival.

Three days after the phone call from Dad, Patricia calls about Tom, who is back in intensive care. She asks me to ask his guides what's wrong. The doctors are puzzled and plan to do another exploratory operation. She's afraid Tom's heart can't survive more surgery. As I meditate, I see three people working on Tom, but rather than being in his hospital bed, he's on an operating table, and they wear robes rather than surgical gowns. One man has his hands on Tom's head, the other on Tom's stomach, while a woman has her hands on Tom's feet.

As I enter the room, the man at Tom's head turns to me and says, "My name is Richard, but my friends call me Rich." He is tall and slender with thin brown hair and long fingers. I find his name odd because all the people I know named Richard are called Dick or Ricky, not Rich. But, I store that thought away for later. They are working on Tom's chakras like a toilet plunger and pull white and gold light through his body from his head to his toes. "Tom has a blockage from his last operation, and we have to keep the energy flowing," Rich explains.

Then I'm back in my bed finishing my meditation and realize that I hadn't introduced myself to them. They had better paranormal manners than I. People on the other side never seemed surprised to see me. It was as if they knew me and knew that I didn't know them.

I tell Patricia about my astral travel to "Richard, but his friends call him Rich," and describe him. "Oh, he was a strong healer in a group I belonged to years ago," Patricia explains. "He worked on Tom when he was first diagnosed with cancer. His name was Richard but everyone called him Rich, and he introduced himself that very way. He died years ago of AIDS."

Well, apparently he is still a strong healer who continues to work on Tom from the other side. Later, Patricia calls again to update Tom's condition. "The doctors found that a portion of his intestinal wall had grown together, which caused a blockage, but it has been repaired and all is well."

After Patricia hangs up the phone, I think *I guess Rich knew what he was doing. He worked on the ethereal body while the doctors figured out what was wrong and fixed the physical body. Makes sense. Can't have one without the other and live in this realm.*

After Patricia tells me Tom's operation was completed, I meditate and find myself beside his bed. Astral traveling to him has become easier and faster. Practice makes perfect? Sitting in a chair, holding Tom's hand, is a woman about seventy-five years of age, her salt-and-pepper hair pulled into a bun. Peering over her spectacles, much like a school librarian, she introduces herself as Margaret. A younger man stands on the other side of the bed and introduces himself as Darrell. They're obviously together from the other side. Margaret doesn't speak, but thinks, "*He's burned out but he'll be okay.*" I hear her thought as clearly as if she had spoken it. This is the first time someone has communicated with me in this manner.

I call Patricia, tell her about Margaret, and describe her.

"Oh, yes. She's an old friend and author, too. In fact she wrote a book about a haunted area on Cape Cod. I have the book here and I'll lend it to you." And that's how I came to read a book by an author I had the pleasure of meeting on the other side.

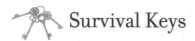 ## Survival Keys

* Feel your connection. We are all connected to the greater oneness of the universe.

* Ask. Anyone can ask for help during trying times and know that the request has been heard and will be answered.

Chapter 22

NASTY FLU, NORMAL CHEMO, OR "CHEMO BRAIN?"

Self-pity is our worst enemy, and if we yield to it,
we can never do anything good in the world.
— Helen Keller (1880–1968)

♥ *Affirmation:* I release any desperation and allow love and balance to fill me.

I have the flu and feel like shit. When feeling this bad after treatment, I've taken my temperature only to see that I'm not running a fever. Today I am. Chills, joint pain, and headache are all part of the therapy roller-coaster ride. Sit back and hold on. The good news is, all rides end.

Three days ago, Peter and I met a cousin (Greeks have many cousins) at an Italian restaurant. I was sipping a lovely glass of wine in the enclosed atrium when she rushed in late, which was fine with me since I no longer have any concept of time (thanks, chemo-brain), gave me a big hug and kiss, then announced that she was late because her boys had the flu. Sirens, lights, and warning bells go off in my head. I should have gotten up and told her I was thrilled to see her but couldn't take a chance on being contaminated by her children through her. But I had already been hugged and kissed. That would be like closing the barn door after the horse has fled. If you weren't personally going through chemotherapy you wouldn't think about things like the flu being passed on to you, but I thought about it. Now, three days later, here I am with a fever of 103 in the Cape Cod Hospital, where I might catch something far worse from some other sick person. My biggest fear, besides losing my life, is that this flu will hold up my chemotherapy, which will result in a prolonged treatment schedule or worse. I don't want to think about *worse* right now. The fate of my tennis friend's sister, who died in an emergency room when left alone with a hydration tube down her throat, pops into my mind again. Peter would never leave me alone, but I made him promise once more, just in case.

"We sent your test results to your Boston doctors and consulted with them. You have the flu, so we're going to give you an antibiotic to head off any secondary infection. Go home, stay in bed, drink plenty of fluids, eat small frequent meals so you won't get nauseated, and we'll see you in five days." The doctor is very kind and answers all my questions about a cold vs. flu vs. chemo aches and fevers. "Tell me what the flu symptoms are like and I'll tell you if I have them," I say, and shiver on the examining table.

"Although colds and flus are both respiratory illnesses, the flu generally is worse than a cold, with symptoms that are more intense." *Of course, but when you're on chemo, they all feel the same — intensely bad! The difference between illness and chemo is fever.* "In the best of health, flu can lead to more serious health issues, like pneumonia. Over-the-counter medications ease symptoms but don't treat the actual virus. So with an already compromised immune system, it's important to immediately seek medical help from a hospital that has a cancer treatment ward," he says, and hands me my prescription.

Now I need to go home and recover, quickly, for my treatment in one week. I'm on a time schedule here. I need to soak in the tub and have a foot massage. That will help, and maybe I'll even whine to Peter through the bubbles. Yes, I'll show him that I really can change, be more like him and whine to get rid of my pent-up aggravation. That should make him proud of me.

While a friend cared for her ill family member she carried alcohol wipes with her and wiped off anything that went into the mouth, including silverware. She also used the wipes after she shook hands with someone. (I hope she waited until they weren't looking.) This sounds like overkill, or the TV show *Monk*, until I think about going back to the emergency room. I only need to be anal retentive about these germs until I get over my treatments and my immune system recovers, along with all the other parts of my body and mind.

In the warm bath, I try to decide which part of my body hurts the most. "I think I've finally lost every hair on my body," I announce to Peter as we massage each other's feet. "Isn't that another full moon?" I ask while running my free hand over my slick, hairless head, still scabby from the latest chemo treatment. Peter shakes his head and mumbles something about not being fixated by the moon like some people he knows. "If it is a full moon again in the same month, that must happen only once in a blue moon," I giggle. "I don't even have any pubic hair left," I whine in a pathetic little voice. I'm feeling very sorry for myself because I feel like shit from the flu and like one of those experimental featherless psycho chickens that pecks itself to death. "I am totally hairless!" After a horrific sneeze, I stare at my hands in disbelief.

"What the hell is that?" Peter asked with a look of horror on his face and pulls his foot back to his side of the tub.

"I think those are my nose hairs," I reply. The mass of tiny black hairs stick to my wet hands. Now I'm totally hairless.

Anyone can get sick from food. Germs abound in public kitchens, but someone in crisis, such as bereavement or divorce, is at a higher risk because stress can compromise an immune system. There is a correlation between stress and illness.

Cold foods prepared in kitchens are often the culprit. Although the kitchen help wear gloves, they are still breathing, talking, laughing, and when sneezing or coughing, cover their mouths with their gloved hands. If you are in crisis, don't eat cold hors d'oeuvres. Hot appetizers right out of the oven are better. When glasses are handed to you, be sure the server is holding the glass from the middle or bottom, not from the drinking area. In other words, don't put your mouth where their fingers might have been. Speaking of fingers, keep them out of your mouth. If you're a nail biter (and being in crisis might make you one if you're not) give it up. Keep your fingers out of your eyes, too.

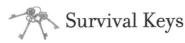 Survival Keys

* Stress from a traumatic experience can manifest as flu-like symptoms with physical pain and weakness. When the spirit is stressed, the body cries out.

* Check your body temperature. If you're running a fever seek medical attention.

* Love and spoil yourself with affirmations, meditations, and whatever gives you joy. This will raise your level of vibration and aid in recovery.

Chapter 23

JUNKIE SYNDROME OR HIGHER VIBRATION

You can't run away from trouble. There ain't no place that far.
—Joel Chandler Harris, *Uncle Remus, His Songs and His Sayings:*
The Folk-Lore of the Old Plantation (1881)

♥ *Affirmation:* I will look into people, as well as at them.

Happy April Fool's Day! The Calends of April, in ancient Rome, always announced stormy weather. History has a way of repeating itself. No third chemo treatment for me on my scheduled appointment. My blood levels are again too low for a treatment. I'm sure the flu didn't help. I hope I can have my second to last treatment the week of the fourth. Well, at least I wasn't all psyched up for my chemo in Boston only to find out I'd have to turn around and go home with my tail between my legs.

Finally, the day before my treatment arrives. I really feel ready, and it's hard to believe that I'm actually happy about this, but I am. Chemo must be melting my brain. We have a fax machine at home, and I've kept track of my blood levels. The faxed results always have ALERT printed on all four sides of the pages in big bold letters. At first this looked pretty scary, but now I've grown accustomed to it. Most people with test results like mine are dying. *Hmm.* The doctors at the Cape hospital called again today and wanted to make sure I wasn't in some kind of medical crisis. Well, I am, but I'm used to it now. No big deal.

I think I've figured out why I'm dizzy all the time. All the chemicals don't help, but it might also be because I've lost all of my body hair, including the tiny hairs inside my ears, which are helpful in maintaining balance. If I sneezed out my nose hairs in the bathtub, I'll bet my ear hairs are gone, too.

The oncologist had warned that the effects of my treatments would be cumulative — each time I'd feel worse, yet on some levels I'm feeling better. I need less nausea medication, and I can do more things outside the house, including gardening. Today, I haven't taken any nausea or pain medicine and I've slept less. At the beginning of this treatment, I'd get out of bed around 10:00, eat breakfast, and go back to bed until 1:00, get up, eat lunch, and get back in bed for a second nap, which lasted until 3:00. At 5:00 I would eat a small dinner and be in bed for the night by 7:30. And that was a good day!

So, I wonder why I feel better now than at the beginning of my treatment. The only explanation I can come up with is my Junkie Syndrome Theory. When a junkie first takes drugs, he gets a certain high; over time, however, he needs a higher dose to get the same high. I think it's the same with chemo drugs. My body has adjusted to them, so it takes more drugs to knock me for the same loop I experienced after the first two sessions. Maybe by my last treatment I won't feel bad at all. Wishful thinking, I'm sure, but like I've said all along, mind over matter. If I don't mind it, it won't matter. Which brings me to my second theory for feeling better despite the statistics — reaching a higher vibration. With all the meditations, dream theory, and positive thinking I've been doing, I've raised my body to a vibration high enough to counteract negativity. It only allows in that which is the highest and best for my body and repels anything else, like nasty side effects.

Peter doesn't agree with my junkie theory because, he says, my blood tests show that my system is extremely distressed. He thinks it's theory number two, higher vibration, all the spiritual meditation and help I've received from my guides. Well, I guess the proof of the pudding is in the eating. My test results say I'm ready to keel over, yet we're going to the Dunbar Tea House for high tea today. I love going out for lunch and not vomiting.

"You look great, Kathy. Look at her, dear! Isn't she glowing? And she's had more treatments than you. See, everything will be fine. There, now, stop crying. Take another tissue."

Doreen has led a weeping patient over to look at me while I'm hooked up to my third treatment. Maybe she had a bad IV nurse or maybe this mad tea party is too much for her, too. Where is that caterpillar with the pipe? Maybe he's hooked up at another chair.

Oh, well, she'll get used to it. We all do. I have no idea why she's crying, but her sadness is contagious. The brightly colored scarf on her head contrasts with her pale skin. She tells me that her doctors didn't get clear margins so the cancer came back ....

Didn't get everything? Has to take treatments again? Peter doesn't fail to see the look of absolute terror on my face. My inner children are totally out of control. Smiling at everyone and nodding in response to this tale of woe, Peter reaches over and places the earphones to his CD player on my head and turns the volume up HIGH. I'm surrounded by music. The Beach Boys' song *Good Vibrations* fills me with joy. My anxiety can't occupy the same space as joy, so anxiety leaves. I can see the weepy patient but can't hear anything she says. In fact I can't even hear the swishing or the ringing in my ears. I smile and nod, and smile and nod.

Lately, I've noticed that when I come in for my treatment, patients tell me their cancer history. Peter and I talked about this after a woman at the check-in desk told me that she had to take Epogen injections because she gained so much weight during chemo that it affected her heart. *What does the heart have to do with Epogen, and how did her heart get damaged by weight gain?!* Those questions did not make me happy. I'm still easily frightened by all this treatment and cancer stuff. I'm familiar with Epogen, a manmade form of protein that helps the body produce red blood cells. I had to give Bluey, my Siamese cat who died six months ago, Epogen shots. But yet another past-life story and lesson has just found new meaning in my present situation. Will the lessons never end?

Maybe when I'm well and strong again I can help others, but not now. Right now I must be my only concern, and my mind must stay peaceful and positive. Chemotherapy treatment centers, like most other recovery centers, are as positive as the personnel who work in them. Yet, for someone who is very sensitive to vibrations and emotions, it's an overload zone. I get saturated with all the emotions of sadness, fear, and pain. I call it free-floating anxiety that always seems to float my way. When it does, Peter turns up the volume on my CD player. Perfect therapy.

Rather than try to remember my questions for Dr. Barkley, I write them down and pin them to my sweater. They are: Is there any way he could ask someone higher up if Deana could do my blood tests, too? Will it hurt the effects of the chemo if I have an occasional glass of wine at dinner? And can I use pure aloe vera gel on my head sores? Dr. Barkley answers, no, no, and yes, then scoots away on his stool.

Ted Williams, the Red Sox baseball player after whom the Ted Williams Tunnel in Boston is named, was leaving the Dana Farber Cancer Institute at the same time I was today. He slowly made his way to a waiting limousine. Despite discomfort from illness and treatment, he smiled for photographers and people asking for autographs. Ted's son wants to have him cryogenically frozen after his death, creating quite a bit of controversy for the rest of the family, who want him buried. After losing Mom to illness, I can empathize with the son. I'd love to have Mom frozen until the day a cancer cure is found. Hell, I'd like to have myself frozen if things don't go well. But I can also sympathize with the rest of Ted's family, too. Having a loved one in suspended animation means no real closure for anyone. How can you find closure with half a goodbye? You'd like to think your loved one is in a better place, with family and friends who have died before her, not in an open-ended frozen dream state where dreams are the reality, as exemplified by Tom Cruise's movie *Vanilla Sky*. But today, Ted Williams was the perfect celebrity, smiling in the face of pain, illness, and cameras. He is a joy. Watching him handle his crisis with dignity renews my confidence.

Survival Keys

✳ Vibrate. Anyone going through any trauma may recovery with less residual negativity by encouraging her body to vibrate at a higher frequency.

✳ Try a new modality. Increasing your frequency can be accomplished with any form or combination of emotional and physical balancing, such as Yoga, meditation, prayer, dream therapy, proper nutrition, and joyful self-expression and experiences.

✳ Walk. A ten-minute walk in the sunshine can accomplish so much that is of a higher physical and emotional vibration. It delivers vitamin D from the sun, which is absorbed through the body, and walking also connects the spirit with nature.

✳ Take care of your spirit, and it will take care of you.

Chapter 24
ADHD and Chemo Brain

*Many of life's failures are people who had not realized
how close they were to success when they gave up.*
— Thomas Alva Edison (1847–1931)

♥ *Affirmation:* I will not give up.

All who wander are not necessarily lost. They could be suffering from "chemo brain," a neurological side effect of chemotherapy that until very recently was dismissed by the medical community. I found chemo brain to be very real, and I described it to my oncologist as a cross between brain constipation, ADD (attention deficit disorder), and Alzheimer's disease. These symptoms are also prevalent in people suffering from depression.

With short-term memory loss and difficulty concentrating, I can't remember where I'm going, how to get there, or why I was even going somewhere, resulting in extreme frustration. I now give myself an extra fifteen minutes to get out of the house because first I can't find my purse, then my keys are missing despite having reminded myself to hang them on the key holder each time I return home. (How do you remind yourself to do something when you can't remember to remind yourself? Yeah — that's chemo brain!) After locating my purse, I realize that in the process, I've put the keys down and lost them again, along with the shopping list I had in my other hand. *Oh, yeah, I pinned the list to my pants pocket. Now I just need those keys and ... my sunglasses! Will I ever get out of this house?*

My solution: Pile everything I need in front of the door the night before so I can't get out of the house without it, and leave the car keys in the car inside the garage. This works as long as Peter is home and can see my pile of stuff in front of the door. He understands my behavior because he has patiently spent hours helping me locate lost items when stress reduced me to tears. The problem is when he comes home before I leave and can't get the door open or falls over the pile. Oh, well, such is life right now.

It's not unusual for me to find myself in front of an open refrigerator with a cup full of hot coffee in my hand and ask myself, "*Why am I here? Do I need something for me or for Peter? Or did I just open the door for the hell of it?*" It's not until I've closed the door and see the coffee cup in my hand that I realize I wanted cream.

My chemo brain is in full swing the days immediately after a treatment. I won't even leave home because I'll forget how to get back, or drive past my street turnoff for the second time, then wonder if it really is my street. That can be frightening.

The positive side to chemo brain is using and working it to your advantage. This is known as selective chemo brain. "Honey did you eat the figs you just washed for me?" Peter calls from the kitchen as he searches for the fruit.

"What figs? Did I buy figs? I don't remember buying figs," I answer from the family room while wiping the last of the fruit off my mouth. Work it while you've got it!

Figs, bran muffins, stool softeners, and laxatives are my new best friends because my brain is not the only part of me that's constipated. Not getting constipated is more important than I thought — as I learned during my first colonoscopy.

"Have you been extremely constipated?" Dr. Fallback asked after the procedure, scheduled because of Mom's colon cancer. After explaining my present predicament he nodded and said, "I thought so. Your colon is healthy and you had no polyps, but there are two small areas in your colon that have developed pouches, similar to diverticulitis, from pushing so hard when using the bathroom. Don't push!"

While we're on the subject of gastroenterologists, we've all heard the TV commercial that insists "four out of five dentists recommend sugarless gum for their patients who chew gum." What did dentist #5 recommend? No gum at all. Recent studies indicate that gastroenterologists agree with that lone dissenting dentist. Folks who chomp on gum throughout the day tend to suck in air, which can cause flare-ups in those who suffer from acid reflux disease. What does that have to do with chemo? We have constant acid reflux. If you want to give your bloated, acidic stomach a break, don't chew gum while in treatment or crisis.

It took some convincing, but Dr. Fallback agreed to do both an endoscopy to examine the upper part of my body, and a colonoscopy; two birds with one stone and only one needle. Hospital policy does not allow for an endoscopy without symptoms, so I gave him one: an extremely upset and painful stomach. Learn to play the hospital policy game and win. I'm setting up an appointment for Peter, too, because everyone should have this kind of checkup every five years. I haven't told him yet. I'll surprise him, later.

Fortunately, chemo brain is not a permanent state of mind, and it too will fade with time. Like the song says, "Don't worry, be happy." Worrying is a useless waste of emotional energy. After rereading this entry, I realize that not worrying is much easier written than done.

ADHD (attention deficit hyperactivity disorder) and ADD (attention deficit disorder) share many of the symptoms of "chemo brain." ADHD has the activity and mood swings not necessarily present in ADD. Trauma can also create these conditions. It's often the natural byproduct of fatigue, depression, and anxiety related to stress, trauma, and treatment. The brain is distracted, the psyche is in crisis mode, and your mind is in overload. Concentration is fleeting. Being distracted and depressed during trauma is annoying but normal.

It's important to remember that this can be a symptom of the bigger problem and can be used as a gauge to monitor progress. As traumatic situations subside, concentration will return. If this condition becomes the straw that breaks the camel's back, seek medical help.

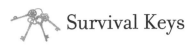 Survival Keys

✳ Remember the word "symptom." Doctors are limited and bound by policy, which dictates what treatment and procedures can be given to patients. If you find that you are in conflict with hospital policy when requesting a test or procedure remember *symptom*. It circumvents policy. Hospital policy is in place for the interest of the hospital, not the patient. A necessary part of any large corporation, policy ensures that the hospital has the finances to be successful.

✳ Become an e-patient. Go online and educate yourself with vocabulary and information so that your doctor and you are speaking the same language.

✳ Describe your symptoms and be sure they're noted in your chart. Documented symptoms are important for getting around the brick wall of hospital policy, and for second opinions and insurance coverage.

✳ Remember this saying: "The pessimist complains about the wind. The optimist expects it to change. And the *leader* adjusts the sails."

✳ Adjust your sails during a crisis with spiritually guided self-advocacy and glide through the storm.

Chapter 25

DOCTOR WITHIN, HEAL THYSELF

Jesus said to them, "Surely you will quote this proverb to me, 'Physician, heal yourself!' Do here in your hometown what we have heard that you do in Capernaum."
— Luke 4:23, The Holy Bible

♥ *Affirmation:* Every cell in my body vibrates with energy and health.

You would think that I'd get a break from all this cancer and psychic stuff on the weekends, but no such luck. I guess my spirit guides don't take the weekends off. I know cancer doesn't. So on this Saturday morning, I'm desperately digging through my bedside drawers for a piece of paper and pencil while repeating the title for a lucid nightmare I've named "The Three Crabs."

I enter through a door into a comfortable, brightly decorated hospital waiting room and greet all the people in the room. I recognize some of them from previous dreams. A happy-looking, tall, dark-haired young woman dressed in a long colorful skirt sits on an ottoman and holds an adorable diapered baby. A woman comes out of her office to my right and introduces herself. "Hi. I'm Dr. Jules." Billy is there, too. He asks, "Why am I here?"

Dr. Jules looks around the room and answers, "We're all here."

As if on cue, three crabs appear, scurry across the floor, and head for the basement door. "Catch them!" I hear someone yell as they dart

140

past me. I give chase and keep them in sight as they scamper down three flights of stairs to the dark tunnels. If they run different directions I'll never find them. My dream has turned into a nightmare.

"Stop!" I yell when they reach the bottom, and I'm shocked when they obey. I scoop them up into a deep clear plastic container filled with water that has materialized in my hand. I gaze at the submerged crabs. They pull in their legs and claws and turn into three pearls. I put a lid on the container and wonder why there are *three* pearls.

Interpretation: This precognitive dream/nightmare deals with medical information and uses the universal symbol for cancer, crabs, which transform into pearls, beauty and perfection through irritation. In my lucid sleep I enter my inner realms and am greeted by all the aspects of myself, but I'm very concerned that there are three crabs, or cancers. I wonder about the accuracy of the information. I had a tumor in my right breast and one lymph node but they were removed. Where is the third crab/pearl? I hope this dream is wrong or it will be a real nightmare in the waking realm. Could I be missing something?

Steve, my old friend from high school and the Ouija board fiasco, calls me on his birthday. We're still close friends. He's the first person I called when Mom died, yet I can't tell him about my health crisis. Maybe I'll tell him when this is all over. Maybe I won't. "I'm doing great!" I lie. "How are you, Steve? Of course I know the date. April 12, Happy Birthday!"

I forgot to call Steve on my birthday this year. If I had remembered, despite my chemo brain, what was I going to say? "Hi, Steve! I just called to tell you that I've driven my doctor completely nuts with an imaginary lump that can't be felt or seen in any tests. And for my birthday I got my third negative mammogram in three months, even though I knew deep inside that it was bogus. So, I'm going back next week to make a bigger pain in the ass of myself until they find something wrong with me to make me happy. I'd go into detail but I can't remember anything because I have chemo brain and had trouble finding the phone to call you. But don't worry! I haven't lost my sense of humor. It's still in my back pocket ... somewhere. Or did I pin it to my shirt?"

I had nothing good to say other than I was still alive, barely, and didn't want to worry Steve, so I chose a white lie over the dark truth.

Truth be told, it's more than that. I can't help myself. I'm such a private person, but there's a reason why it's good to keep in contact with people who don't know what I'm going through: I can pretend to be normal. For those few minutes while I speak with them, Kathy in Cancerland is gone and the old Kathy is back, laughing about old times and planning for the future.

When I taught the profoundly emotionally disturbed, I used to tell my students that if they could act normal they could be normal. I often saw their transformation when we went to restaurants for lunch or on field trips. We get so used to our limitations controlling us that we forget how to be happy and free. Sometimes you have to "Fake it till you make it." It's another life lesson from the past that touches my present and molds my future. Amazing!

Happy Anniversary, Mom! Today is your day. I remember this day well and the memory is murder. It feels like only yesterday, yet so much has happened since that full moon during your hour of souls. I need to say that I'm glad you're not alive to see the bumpy road I've traveled this past year, because it probably would have killed you, but I know that you know. Even though you went on ahead of me to the other side, I've felt you beside me every step of the way, and I'm reminded of the poem "Footprints in the Sand," which I received as a Christmas card from an astute friend. It made me realize that when I was seeing only one set of footprints in the sand rather than two, it was because I was being carried through my darkest hour.

Mom, I know you and God have been here to carry me. I just want you to know that despite all that's happened to me, I know the negative aspect of this challenge is only temporary. I see this as a learning experience that has given me depth of character and empathy I could never have developed without it. I am grateful for all the love and support I've received from everyone, here on earth and from on your side.

You know how important silver linings are to me. Well, if there's a silver lining to your suffering it's that it taught me how to get though my suffering with dignity and grace. Much of what we learned together during your crisis has helped me now.

I've still been looking for a distributor of the hydrazine sulfate that I found for you to reduce weight loss when you were too ill to eat, but all the leads have dried up.

In a few days I'll be done with chemo. Now, I know what you went through with your reports. Talk about emotional torture. No — I really don't know what you went through; my report didn't tell me my condition was terminal, that cancer had metastasized throughout my body, and that I had only a few weeks to live. I'm sorry I wasn't with you for that diagnosis, but looking back, I think it might have killed me if I had been. Yet you were so strong, saying, "Death is the only way we get off this planet. No one leaves here alive." I hope I have that same strength to draw on when my time comes, and half the grace you exhibited.

I love and miss you so much. See you soon, in my dreams.

There is something in the healing process called anniversary reactions: responses that occur following reminders of a loss. Linda, my Indian/wolf therapist, said these reactions are not setbacks in the grieving process but rather big steps forward that we take by not getting stuck in denial.

Grief is a part of life.

Feel it,

Respond to it,

And move on.

I've experienced how some people in certain religions respond publicly with special services for families and friends at different intervals throughout the grieving process. My way is a private letter that I've just set ablaze and will send to Mom by purified smoke.

Survival Keys

* Know that anniversary reactions can be a way
of healing during and after any crisis such as
bereavement, abuse, or residual emotions related to
a trauma.

* Convert deeply buried emotions into written words
and bring them to the surface from deep within the
psyche. It manifests them in a safe environment
where they can be overcome. Read them aloud or
silently before burning them to erase them forever.
Emotions may still surface, but those particular
words are gone forever. Words and memories are
powerful. So is fire.

Chapter 26

MORE TREATMENT?
WHEN ENOUGH IS ENOUGH

Inner guidance is the missing piece to our Life Puzzle.
Dreams fit our pieces together.
— Kathleen O'Keefe-Kanavos

♥ *Affirmation:* My emotions calm themselves as I realize
all is well in the moment.

It's been three weeks since my last treatment, and now it's time for my last mid-treatment blood test. My Cape vein angel arrives with her smile and tiny needle. "You look so well. Will this week be your last chemo?" she wisely asks to distract me.

"I believe so. My doctor talked to me about a second chemotherapy treatment called Taxol, but I've decided not to take it because the California doctor said it didn't respond to the CSRA tests." I tell her about Tumor Kill typing and how most insurance companies won't pay for the CSRA tests. "Taxol has major side effects and is only guaranteed to hold off cancer recurrence for five years. I think it would be groundless overkill."

"You would think the insurance companies would find it less expensive to do the correct chemo on someone just once rather than multiple times until it works, not to mention the cost of the side effects of the treatment," she says, and quickly removes the needle.

"Taxol is a very strong drug that's still in the testing stage. I don't want to be tested with something that I'm not sure will even work for me. I can just see me serving the tennis ball with a numb hand from neuropathy, and have my racket fly out of my hand and hit the net player in the head. No, thanks."

She gives me a big goodbye hug and said she hoped she wouldn't see me anymore. "But if you need me, you know where I am."

This was a special moment. It was my first "end" — the first "last time" for anything dealing with treatment, and that was a turning point. I walk out of the clinic like I'm walking on air. I hope that's a good omen. Tomorrow will tell. I feel like a downed gladiator in the Roman arena waiting for that reprieve from Caesar.

Thumbs down! My blood levels are still too low for my last chemo. I am so sick of this. I'm sick and tired of being sick and tired. *Calm down. This is just another bump in the road of Cancerland. Shhh, Shhh. Remember, mind over matter, mind over matter.* I'll meditate to pull up my blood counts. Another Tiny Bubbles dream would help.

I need to look on the bright side of everything to keep myself motivated and positive, so my closing positive thought for this entry is: This could be much worse. Being a sensitive (my description of myself to avoid the word "psychic"), I'm very sensitive to drugs and at any time could have had a very bad reaction to the treatments and ended up in an emergency room late at night, like my tennis friend's sister, and dead. I think I just made myself feel better? After rereading that cheerful (NOT!) entry, I think I need to stop writing.

Finally! I'll have my last chemo treatment on the last day of the month, April 30. Overall, I'm a month late finishing treatment, but better late than never. Done is *done!*

On the way to the hospital, I don't even need to whine anymore. Peter just pulls into "our gas station" and patiently waits for me. Then I immediately start sipping my hot herbal tea from a child's heat-reactive flashing sippy cup that I found in K-Mart. On the tenth floor of the Dana-Farber, I run to the bathroom first, then soak my arm in the sink. The next stop is Dr. Barkley's office on the ninth floor for blood test results, and back up to the tenth floor for treatment. "Is that cup flashing?" Dr. Barkley asks, peering over his glasses.

"Yes, it's a child's spill-proof sippy cup, perfect for my hot tea," I answer, holding it up for his inspection. "The heat from the tea activates the flashing flowers."

He says I never cease to amuse him, and by the time I finish my treatments, I've started a new trend — there are flashing sippy cups everywhere, happy winking flowers.

With my chemo brain, I often get confused as to which floor I'm on — yeah, it's that bad.

"Peter, where are we?" I'll ask inside the elevator trying to decide which button to push.

The look of shock on his face concerns me more than being lost between two floors. Oh, well, so what? Mind over matter. I don't mind it, so it doesn't matter. Blame chemo brain and move down one place setting at the mad tea party. The crazy party is almost over.

Oh, happy days! My blood counts are up. I'm off to the elevators to the ninth-floor infusion room, hopefully for the last time in my life. "I want to see you in one month, so make an appointment at the front desk before you leave," Dr. Barkley says as he hugs me before I run out the door. *I'll call the front desk and make that appointment, later. Right now, I'm outta here!* Peter can hardly keep up with me. The race is on. I'm heading for the finish line. I can see it.

Deana, my IV nurse, greets me with a big hug and smile. "Last treatment!" she says in an excited whisper. My bags of many colors still looked like an abstract Christmas tree from a Dr. Seuss book. All I need now is for Thing One and Thing Two to pop out from behind a curtain and raise hell because everything is progressing too well. My earphones are on, and I'm listening to my soothing meditation tape when the psychiatrist walks up with Doreen. I had anticipated seeing her one last time and have brought her a box of Belgian truffles. She has been an incredible help to me during all this.

"Thank you for your help and understanding," I yell. Shocked faces peer at me from around the room. I turn down the volume. We discuss

what a long emotional trip this had been and how far I've come from
that frightened, angry person curled up in a ball to guard my arms.
We all had a good laugh, and it is during this laughter that the tide
turns. I look at a dire situation through eyes that see humor, laughing
at myself and with myself. Progress!

Peter and I decided last night that if I have this last treatment
today we would celebrate by going to a fancy restaurant in Boston,
anywhere I wanted to go. I choose Jimmy's Harborside on the docks of
South Boston. I'm looking forward to this dinner celebration despite
my lack of appetite. I've perfected pretending to eat in public, now,
and will continue to fake it till I make it. Just the thought of me in a
fancy restaurant like a normal person makes me smile. I settle into the
infusion chair for the last time and savor my thoughts like a fine wine.

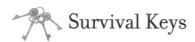 ## Survival Keys

* Realize that conventional treatment is a gift from
  God administered by physicians.

* Reach balance. Over-treatment is overkill, and can
  be as bad as or worse than no treatment at all. The
  patient, by going within and seeking inner guidance
  through dreams, meditations, and prayer, should
  be the one to say when enough is enough, even if it
  goes against the advice of the doctors. Listen to your
  medical doctor, but remember that you must make
  the final decision. Consult your physician-within.

Chapter 27

CELEBRATE THE GOOD TIMES

Happiness is a perfume you cannot pour on others
without getting a few drops on yourself.
— Ralph Waldo Emerson (1803–1882)

♥ *Affirmation:* The soul always knows what to do to heal itself. The challenge is to silence the mind. I will overcome the challenge of silencing my mind and listen to my spirit.

Jimmy's Harborside has fantastic views of Boston Harbor. Peter called and requested a special table. Our waiter is always there when we need him and gone when we don't. My glass of red wine does its magic. The oily legs slide down the side of the glass and dance in the reflection of the candlelight. I drink with caution because keeling over on the floor would not be a great ending to a special day. Dr. Barkley said wine with dinner would actually be good for me. I love it when we're of the same mind.

After our little toast to the future, I feel hungry for the first time in months. The magic in the wine must be working because, if anything, I should feel worse after this last treatment. Maybe I should have had a glass of wine before each meal throughout my whole treatment. The plate was empty. I had finished all of my baked stuffed lobster.

We toast again to this treatment down and one left to go: radiation. But right now I don't want to think about that. Let's bask in the joy of this moment. I'm done. I'm done. *Thank you God, guides, and angels for helping me get through this ordeal alive. After this wonderful dinner I'll go home and have a nice sleep, no nightmares or important dreams. I've already said thank you, so I'd prefer not to chat tonight. I just want to sleep.*

Well, I slept well last night because the communication came *before* I fell asleep. It's uncanny how my guides hear my requests and respond accordingly. My nightly meditation turned very fishy last night.

Rather than the meditation ending after God's golden light fills all seven of my chakras and the seven goblets become one, from which I drink, a voice says, "Wait."

Seven pieces of swordfish cut into triangles cover each chakra. A dandelion with a big yellow flower is placed on the piece of fish on my fourth, or heart, chakra. Then a large chalice appears in my hand, and I drink from it before falling asleep.

Interpretation: The color gold is the higher self, and 7 is a sacred number, a combination of three (heaven) plus four (earth), equaling a mystical relationship of perfect order and the dual nature of balance. A triangle is the symbol for fire, which purifies. Swordfish is a play on words, but my guides knew I would figure it out. The "sword of justice" divides truth from falsehood and is constructive or destructive depending on the wielder of the sword. Fish is the Christ within, and swordfish cut into triangles symbolizes purity and balance to empower the seven chakras. The dandelion flower may be another play on words — a dandy lion. In ancient Christian symbolism the lion represents Jesus. So putting the dandelion on the heart chakra gives way to the idea of lionhearted. Blossoms symbolize new life and fruits of the spirit. The dandelion is also my flower, given to me by my guides in a previous meditation.

My guides and angels just armed me with more gifts for round three of my treatments.

Mayday, Mayday, I think I'm crashing! Rather than ribbons around a Maypole, I have buzzing around my head. My ears are ringing and my balance is off. I don't feel particularly nauseous, but rather like a gassed bug. Great! Now this experience has given me empathy for bugs. I'm going to be a Buddha by the end of my treatments. If I feel like this one day after my last chemo infusion, what will I feel like in ten days? I'll know soon enough.

The good news is that I don't feel nauseated or want anyone to shoot me like I did after the first chemotherapy treatment four months ago. So, how much worse can it be when I finally crash? Never mind — don't wanna go there!

Well, today is without a doubt the worst of all my days. It's May 9, my crash day and Mother's Day. I'm crashing *and burning*. Yeah! Talk about adding more insult to injury. I'm so depressed I'm moving in slow motion.

When I turned on the news this morning, I soon realized that I'd completely lost track of time and holidays. I always took Mother's Day for granted and never noticed how packed the airways were with mommy stuff. It's like never noticing how many food commercials there are on TV at night until you go on a diet. I've gone into hiding. Mother's Day is everywhere. For the first time in my life, I'm on the outside looking in, and I hate it!

It's been two weeks and two days since my last chemotherapy, and despite the Mother's Day fiasco I'm either starting to crash or beginning to recover. I've never felt this tired and sluggish. I thought this last crash/recovery would be different from all the others, so, rather than rest, I went to the TJ MAXX department store to shop. This was a bad idea because I'm about to faint. I don't even have the energy to walk back to the bathroom I so desperately need. The last time I had a difficult decision to make concerning this very same predicament was when I brought Mom here after her colon surgery. History keeps repeating itself. I must make an important choice: Walk back very slowly to that same bathroom and hope I don't pass out on the way, or turn around now and, while holding onto whatever I can for support, make my way to the car and go home to my own bathroom. After careful consideration, I decide to "hold it" and head for home. Alas, although I am done with my treatments, they are not yet done with me.

I've become anorexic, and hope that this side effect will pass, too. Even wine doesn't help me anymore. Again, this disease has given me sympathy and empathy for another group of people I never believed I'd ever have anything in common with anorexics.

Saturday night we went to dinner with friends, and the menu gave me an anxiety attack. My palms began to sweat as my heart raced and fluttered. In the past I responded to food with glee; now I feel only dread.

"Kathy, I'm going to order two appetizers and eat the second one as my main meal," Shirley says with a sideways glance at me. I guess my anxiety showed more than I thought. Was it my bulging eyes or my sweaty upper lip?

"Great idea. I will, too," I say. "And I think I'll order something I've never tried before so I won't be disappointed if I don't like it." Everything still tastes metallic, so maybe I'll just eat the fork here and take the spoon home for later. That should be different.

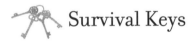 Survival Keys

* Allow change. Crisis changes not only the person but also the world around her.

* Know that you will often feel like your body and mind are working against you with anxiety attacks and constant changes in perspective concerning life. What was once spontaneous fun becomes a burdensome obligation.

* Form new habits. By changing habits, new, joyful patterns can take the place of "tried and true" patterns that no longer work.

Part III

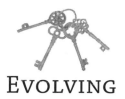

EVOLVING

Chapter 28

RADIATION, TATTOOS, AND CONCENTRATION CAMPS

*A hot bath! I cry, as I sit down in it; and again, as I lie flat,
a hot bath! How exquisite a pleasure, how luxurious,
fervid and flagrant a consolation for the rigours,
the austerities, the renunciations of the day.*
— Rose Macaulay (1881–1958)

♥ **Affirmation:** The more grateful I am, the more reasons I find to be grateful.

It's been three weeks since my last chemo, and I feel relatively human again. I'm preparing physically and mentally for radiation by researching it. The National Cancer Institute defines radiation therapy as the use of an energy called ionizing radiation to kill cancer cells and shrink tumors. It injures or destroys cancer cells in the area being treated by damaging their genetic material, which prevents the cells from either growing or replicating.

It won't be as bad as chemo, but that's not saying much.

My sister-in-law gave me the phone number for the R.A. Bloch Cancer Hotline. A friend of hers used it when he was diagnosed with prostate cancer. His hotline mentor helped him through every step of his treatment, including radiation. That's what I need — a mentor! I still haven't found a helpful book, so a real person will do.

"The hotline finds a mentor your age who has survived a similar cancer," the volunteer explains when I call. Although I've read medical information, I want to know what to expect emotionally, and get any hints someone might have to put my mind at ease. Will it be as fatiguing or painful as chemotherapy? Will it give me mood swings? Will my tiny hairs fall out again? I have questions that I don't even know how to formulate because I don't know enough about this treatment to frame them. But I'm as happy as a pig in mud to finally be at this stage of treatment. I'm moving right along.

"Thank you for your information. We'll find someone for you to speak with. They'll probably call you at home tonight." I thank her and look forward to the conversation.

"Hi, thiz Jenny callin' from The Cancer Hotline. I'm looking fur Kathy O'Keefe– Kannan, no, Kavia, is that right?"

"Don't worry," I reassure her. "It sounded Greek to me the first time, too." Thus begins my education on radiation therapy by Jenny in Tennessee with her strong southern drawl. I recognize her accent from the military base at Fort Campbell, Kentucky, where I continuously asked my new friends, "Please spell it. I can't understand you." It must have been more training for my trauma today, twenty-some years later.

"Radiation's a breeze compared to chemo. Treatment's 'bout six weeks long, five days a week. You get weekends 'n' holidays off. Worst parts not showerin' the whole time."

"Why couldn't you shower?" I repeat to be sure I'd heard correctly.

She explains that at the "mapping session" they draw on you with magic markers and don't want you to wash them off. So she carefully bathed in the sink. "It was only fur six weeks, so I didn't miss showerin' too much. 'Course, they might do thangs different where yur from, but that's how they do 'em here in Tennessee."

No showers for six weeks. That sounds like torture, but if that's the way things must be, I won't complain, much.

"If you want to speak with me again, call the hotline and ask for me by name."

I thank Jenny and hang up. At least I feel armed with some intelligent information for my radiation oncologist's meeting. I won't look shocked when told not to bathe for six weeks. I won't be caught off guard.

Two days later I drive myself to my first radiation therapy meeting while Peter sits in the back seat with his iced leg hanging over the headrest. While boxing my rose bushes, he'd had an accident with our electric hedge trimmer: he hit his knee with it. My bushes don't have buds or flowers, but Peter has a limp and stitches. I also thought about last night's long and wonderful bubble bath that would have to last me six whole weeks. Peter even climbed into the tub and hung his leg over the edge.

You'd think that, after all the times I traveled to my treatments, I'd know the route by heart. Actually, the car should be able to drive itself, but I can't remember much of the previous trips because I was too nervous before the treatments to focus, and afterward I had major chemo brain and couldn't concentrate. So, today we're the quintessential ship of fools with Chemo Brain driving and Limpy acting as the back-seat driver: Laurel and Hardy in treatment.

"Dan, if your wife had cancer, who would you send her to for radiation treatment?" Peter had asked our oncologist friend in Miami over the phone after my diagnosis. "Dr. Harold," he answered without hesitation. "He doesn't usually take new patients. Tell him I sent you." Dr. Harold's infectious joy for life permeates the examining room. I like him instantly and feel my fears melt away under the warmth of his smile.

"Your first appointment will be an ultrasound to see how deep the radiation beams can go without damaging extra tissue, especially the lungs and heart. A few days later, with that information to guide me, we'll do the mapping," Dr. Harold said, as much to me as to the two interns flanking him and taking copious notes.

"What if there's *something* in the area? You know, what if some leftover cancer shows up?" I ask the nurse nonchalantly as she helps me dress. The question shows how frightened I still am. *Something* could still get me! But if something is there, do I really want to know, or would I rather hide in ignorance? Ignorance can be bliss. I need some bliss.

"There shouldn't be anything there," the nurse says gently, sensing my fear. I'll bet she deals with this often, but it's still new to me. "Between the surgery and chemo everything is gone. This ultrasound isn't for problems, it's strictly for measurement."

Get a hold of yourself and stop this mind babble. You're going to make yourself crazy or at the very least raise your blood pressure, the parent within me chides.

Dr. Harold reenters the room with the two previous interns and a new one. My mapping session will be done at the Brigham and Women's' Hospital on the lower second floor. Nuclear medicines are housed in basements surrounded by lead walls, resulting in no cell phone service. That thought didn't help my blood pressure. If they need lead walls to keep escaped rays from affecting the outside world, what the hell are we doing down here? *Shhh!* I have a new respect for doctors and interns who subject themselves to radiation on my behalf.

Dr. Harold explains that a mapping consists of two parts — calibrating radiation beams to target the surgery area of my right breast, and tattoos, so the technicians can line up the machine and beams correctly for each day's treatment.

"I'll be marked with magic markers and tattooed!" I repeated while smiling to keep my sense of humor. "Plus, I can't bathe for six weeks. I'm going to be a stinky jigsaw puzzle."

Silence! Everyone in the examining room, doctors and nurses alike, freezes and looks flabbergasted. Before the pregnant pause could drag on too long, I tell them about my phone conversation with Jenny, the Cancer Hot Line woman in Tennessee.

"This is not Tennessee. We do things differently here, and the radiation technicians would greatly appreciate you bathing at least once a day," Dr. Harold replies with a broad smile. The others in the room nod in agreement and stare down at their feet, trying not to laugh.

Was Jenny pulling my leg? Surely not! Maybe they really do things differently down there. I'll bet this story will be circulated with glee at intern parties. I can already hear it: "Remind me not to intern in Tennessee without a nose clip." But it's amazing how much you can enjoy a bath if you think it will be your last for a while.

Two days later, while lying on the mapping table with my arm bent precariously over my head for the best radiation alignment angle, I'm observed through an elevated glass window by my radiologist and specialists. Despite someone's attempt to make L2, as the basement level of Brigham and Women's hospital is known, cheery, it reminds me of the air raid bunkers in Europe. That's befitting since I'm at war. I have to fight the urge to ask a man getting on the elevator as I got off, "Excuse me, what level of hell is this?" Little did I know that the memories would get much worse. *Mind over matter. I am number one. I am important. Nothing is more impor —.* My physical therapy homework of "walking the wall" recaptured my arm's full range of motion. Without it, I'd be in real pain right now.

Artificial intelligence rules the room. Massive machines, operated from behind large plate glass windows, move gracefully around me. They stop occasionally to cross communicate with beeps and buzzes before continuing on their circular path around my body like misshapen planets moving through time and space. Classical music could make this a machine ballet. "We're almost done, Kathy. Then a technician will come in to tattoo you."

Tattoo me! That shocks me out of my meditation. *Oh, yeah! I remember.* My thoughts wandered to my nanny, Tanta Martha, in Germany, the Dachau concentration camp in Munich, and the tattoo on her arm ... .

The Dachau death camp had been only eighteen kilometers from my high school, so my church group went there for a field trip — TO HELL!

Above the huge black gates the words ARBEIT MACHT FREI greeted me. After reading WORK MAKES YOU FREE, did Tanta Martha and thousands of other prisoners wonder, "If I work hard will I be free from memories of loved ones missing, dead, and experimented on?"

Yeah, right! I thought as I walked through the same gates in the same footsteps as those thousands of prisoners and my nanny ... into hell on earth.

Thick as Jell-O is the only way to describe the air in the death camp. I found breathing and walking through it almost impossible as I made my way across the barren entryway to the first of the thirty-four barracks buildings, one of which had housed my nanny. My friends had followed our tour guide in a different direction. I ignored her warning to stay with the group and followed my instincts to an area to which I felt pulled. The camp was fenced in, so how could I get lost? This particular barrack was long and narrow with parallel wooden communal bunk beds that extended the length of the space. The room contained an absence of light. Rather than reflecting light off the floor or through doorways, it devoured light like a black widow spider consuming a butterfly, and left behind grayness that blended with shadow. There weren't even dust particles dancing in the air. Nothing danced here. This place seemed to possess its own gravity. Out of the corner of my eye I saw a foot or shoe protrude from a corner, but when I looked directly at the spot it was empty. A shuffling noise to my right reassured me that my friends from my disastrous Ouija party had come to rescue me from my wild imagination. With a sense of relief, I tore my eyes from the shadowy corner and moved in the direction of the noise to greet them, but there was no one there, just more gray emptiness mixed with a damp cold I hadn't noticed earlier.

I'm outta here! I sprinted toward the doorway but was startled by a small face that stared up at me from the dark lower level of a bunk bed. The face pulled back into the shadows and disappeared as soon as it had my undivided attention.

I ran from the building and toward the sound of my friends only to come face to face with a large shower room flanked by four smaller ones — gas chambers. I saw what appeared as a daydream: prisoners disrobing and anxiously but resolutely entering the showers, holding hands, knowing this would be their last human touch because they were going to die. As the doors closed I saw myself inside, throwing my hands up in an act of finality that said, "God, cleanse me of this world," and welcomed the deadly gas with deep, deliberate breaths. Death, not work, was freedom from this hellhole.

"Kathy, why are you here alone," our guide asked after she'd located me back on the bus.

"I saw bones in the oven and I had to get out of there," I replied. I sat in the last seat of the bus to be sure nothing could sneak up behind me.

"That's impossible. Those ovens were cleaned out long ago. The prisoners were buried in mass graves outside the camp behind the showers because of the coal shortage. It was too expensive to burn them," she replied in her heavy German accent.

I saw and heard people where there should have been no one, saw bones in ovens that were supposedly cleaned, and walked through Jell-O. I wanted to go home. If this terrible place affected me like this after twenty minutes, what had it done to those poor prisoners who were here for a lifetime, like Tanta Martha? The faces I saw in the dark corners and the nightly marching "ghost soldiers" in Berlin proved that just because people are dead doesn't mean they are gone.

The blinding overhead lights of the radiation mapping room shocks me out of my scary memories and back to my dismal reality. A technician appeared beside me. "You can put your arm down now," she said. "Those lights are bright, but I need them to see where to put the tattoos since they're so tiny, just the size of a pinhead, and will fade in time. They're in blue ink so we won't confuse them with your freckles."

I squinted and tried to shield my eyes from the glare, but my fingertips were numb from lack of circulation. She deposited droplets of blue ink in strategic places on my chest, then gave them a quick poke with a needle. The discomfort was minimal. She helped me into a sitting position and readjusted my gown.

"The doctor's office will call with the date for your first treatment close to the beginning of June. It takes ten days for the calibrations to come in," the nurse said.

Next, I went upstairs to the ninth floor of the Dana-Farber and saw Dr. Barkley and Dr. Kritchen for my first one-month post-chemotherapy and surgery checkups.

I've been prescribed Tamoxifen, and will start it now rather than after radiation therapy. Tamoxifen is hormone therapy. Women on Tamoxifen for five years have 40 to 50% reduction in recurrence. Now, should I or should I not make friends during radiation?

Survival Keys

* Feel that you are not alone. Upon hearing a diagnosis
  of severe illness, many people feel devastated,
  confused, and alone. Even in our darkest hour—we
  are never alone.

* Connect. Crisis mentors are people from the
  trenches of experience who offer reassurance by
  simply existing. They are thrivers helping survivors.

Chapter 29

RADIATION FRIENDS

Living your life's dreams is a life well lived.
— Kathleen O'Keefe-Kanavos

♥ *Affirmation:* I choose love, joy, and freedom, open my heart, and allow wonderful things to flow into my life.

"I'm Laura, your radiation nurse. Choose any locker for your clothing, but they don't have locks, so take your purse with you. The gowns and two changing rooms are behind you. If you used deodorant today please use a towelette to wipe it off." She points to a blue plastic box. "Deodorant, body creams, and perfumes can affect the radiation beams."

I imagine wild beams bouncing off a deodorant particle, hitting me in the eye and blinding me. *Really! Stop imagining things like that,* my inner parent chides.

The nurse leaves me with my savage thoughts. Since the guides gave me the number two as my number, I choose it and then enter the waiting room.

"Hi, my name is Becky. Is this your first day, too? Don't you just love these gowns?" She twirls the tie suggestively and strikes a pose. "Do these make a fashion statement or what? I think I'll wear mine home in the car and flash people on the highway."

We bonded. My previous decision not to make friends during treatment flew out the window, figuratively speaking, of course, because there are no windows down here. That no-friend decision was based on memories of my waitressing days at the officer's club at Fort Devens. Officers discussed how they never bonded with new soldiers who replaced dead ones. It was an emotional necessity for survival and sanity. I was thinking along those same lines, but before I realized what had happened, Becky and I were comparing notes on our situations as if we were talking about our flower gardens. She knew exactly what I was going through because she was, too, right here, right now, with me. We bonded like war buddies sharing a foxhole. My need for a comrade overrode my fear of loss.

When Becky switched her yearly mammograms to the Faulkner Hospital, a six-centimeter tumor was found in her left breast, resulting in a mastectomy. "But I'm not going to have reconstructive surgery. Only one boob doesn't bother me. My husband still loves me, so why go through that pain?" My sister-in-law said the same thing years ago. I don't know what I would do if I had to have my breast removed. The idea scares me, but Becky's story reinforces Life Lesson #2: Go somewhere reputable for mammograms!

Her chemo was the same as mine, Adriamycin/Cytoxan, followed with Taxol, which she discontinued because it made her sick and her fingers and toes numb from neuropathy. Her tumor is non-hormone receptive, so she's not taking Tamoxifen.

"Kathy, we're ready for you." I walk past monitoring screens. I would be watched. I recline on the table with my arm held in the same blood-draining position as during the mapping, breasts secured with white netting. I looked like a bizarre Renoir painting: *Therapy in the Nude*. Then the technicians scurry out of the room.

"Call us if you need us. We can hear and see you on the monitors."

Are they all leaving me? Do I have to stay in here alone? I feel a fight-or-flight reaction. *Shouldn't I throw off this stuff and view this room over their shoulder, too? If this place is so dangerous, what am I doing here? What if I explode like a piece of popcorn?*

Shhh, my inner parent said. *People do this every day and you are not alone. Your spirit guides are here. Surround yourself with Reiki energy and meditate. Say, "Only that which is of the highest and best for me may affect my body in a positive manner."* So I do, as the sounds of whining, beeping, and conversation fade into the background.

"See you tomorrow, Becky. It was a breeze — only took a few minutes inside the room," I reassure her as she's led into the radiation room with that deer in the headlights look.

In the main waiting area Peter had been talking to Becky's husband Jack. "I might not be able to stay down here with you each time, Bunny, because I can't get any phone service for my conference calls," Peter says, an apologetic look on his face.

"That's fine. I made a friend. I won't be lonely. One treatment down, thirty-five to go."

"Yes, suicide is an option, but let's keep it as a last one, because it's permanent! Save it for after you've tried everything else," I heard as I put my things in locker number two. The weekend was over!

The nurses weren't around, and Linda, who had almost completed her treatment, was leading the discussion. "Does anyone know of a successful and painless way to commit suicide?"

That question took me back to my own mental discussions with my inner selves and guides concerning Team Earth and the rules of suicide. The discussion seemed like yesterday and a lifetime ago, rather than four months. I know where all this is coming from; I just don't know where it's going. It reminded me of another time, fifteen years ago in Florida.

She was the young, tall, blond, beautiful wife of a prominent doctor — with an inoperable brain tumor. She decided to have a wonderful goodbye party before taking her own life, dressed in a designer gown bought especially for the occasion. Donna had the perfect party, was the perfect hostess, and attempted suicide with an overdose of pills that didn't go perfectly. It put her loved ones in the precarious situation of helping her die. This could have caused the end of their practices and futures in the medical field. Simple deaths from overdoses of sleeping pills or pain medication are strictly Hollywood, not reality. Suicide is a tricky business. People don't die easily, even by their own hand. It's human nature to fight for every single precious moment of life.

Suicide is serious. You can't call back the bullet, literally or figura-tively, and it can be contagious. Desperate people make suicide pacts so they don't have to face the unknown alone. Some of the people in this room might qualify as desperate, so as gently but sternly as possible, I explain this to the group without letting them know what I knew about life on the other side. If this is a decision that's been seriously contemplated by someone who knows when to throw in the towel, then I don't want to change her mind; however, I also don't want to see someone give up and lose out to fear. We're all afraid right now and that's okay. It's normal.

Changing back into my clothes, I gaze into the dressing room mirror and am surprised by the reflection staring back. I look good. I really do! But what impresses me most is the look deep in my eyes — a depth of confidence previously absent. "Whooo are yooou?"

Who am I today? Am I done morphing into someone new or am I still changing? Like Alice, will I suddenly start growing or shrink away? I step closer and stare at myself for a minute to see exactly what it is about that gaze that seems so different. I see myself blush from embarrassment. I've invaded a stranger's space. "What is it that's so different about you?" I ask the person in the mirror, and then I see it! Fear has been replaced by confidence. Fear is still there somewhere, but has been pushed back and out of sight. Whenever I see immo-bile patients wheeled here for more treatment, I feel fear pushing its way to the surface, but I never let it break through. An invisible hand forces it back down into the depths of my being.

Kathy, send that person love and energy, because nothing ever just happens. You were meant to meet here and be one with her, if only for a moment. When our eyes meet for that split second, I wonder if we are ships passing in the night or old souls recognizing each other. And are we exactly where we need to be at this moment? Our ships are connected by the cross-waves of time and circumstance, even in the darkest hour of night's fog. Nothing is an accident.

I've become both the ultimate observer and participant in my pro-cess of change. If this is my new self-made reality, how far down the rabbit hole will I go? And do I have any control over the depth of my fall? The eyes answered, "*It's your reality. How far do you want to go? What do you want to do when you get there? Remember: if you don't mind it, it won't matter.*"

As I turn from the mirror, I realize it's Friday. My second week of radiation therapy is completed. Other than our discussion groups, it's been pretty repetitious. Actually, the best days were when sessions ran late and more women were added to our discussions. Before we head home today, Peter and I will pick up my Florida tennis partner, Jill, from the airport. Despite the dire details of my treatments, she still wants to spend a long weekend with me.

It's Saturday afternoon naptime, even though I got up at 10:00 a.m. Things are floating before my eyes, and my ears ring so badly it's downright scary. It sounds like I have bugs in them. Is this going to get louder with each radiation treatment? I must be hallucinating, going blind, or both. What's weird is Baby Cakes seems to be batting at things floating in front of my eyes. My cat is infected with my hallucinations. Is the radiation seeping off me and onto him when he wraps his paws around my neck? Alarmed for Baby, I stop petting him.

"What's that buzzing sound? Is the radio on?" Peter asks, coming up to tuck me in.

Can the ringing in one's ears and a hallucination be shared by people and animals? Peter opens the drapes for a better look. The room is full of bees!

"Jill!" I yell as I shake out the bedcover full of previously unseen bees. How did I walk across the bee-covered floor without being stung?

Jill had apiaries in Pennsylvania and sold honey, so she knew bees. "Let's see if they fly outside," Jill said, opening the sliding glass door to the balcony. Like the Pied Piper of Hamlin the bees follow her onto the porch, take an immediate right turn, and fly straight up to the chimney top where they reenter the house.

"You have a swarm of honeybees with a queen in the chimney," Jill explains, peering cautiously up the chimney. "They won't attack unless you threaten the queen."

"Make them go away!" I say from beneath the safety of my bedcovers, coming out long enough to flick another bee onto the floor with its hive mates. "Where's Peter?"

"He limped away, fearful of being stung on his good leg," Jill echoes from the chimney.

As if on cue, Peter reappears with a fly swatter and a can of wasp spray that shoots a stream of insecticide up to ten feet. He begins to swat and spray like an athlete playing a bizarre game of skeet shooting and flyswatter tennis. Walls dripped with insecticide and writhing bees.

"That might make them angry." Jill calls from the safety of a far corner.

We tape paper bags across the fireplace like a patchwork quilt, and then call pest control. "Take your nap, Bunny. I'll handle this." Peter must have mistaken the look of relief on my face as respite from the swarm, but it was reassurance. I'm not hallucinating from radiation.

Just as I'm dozing off, Peter reenters the bedroom with another sinister-looking canister. "What's that?"

"A bug bomb," he chuckles, and heads for the taped-up chimney. "Bug specialists don't work on weekends, and we can't "bother" the bees because they're an endangered species. We'd have to wait until Monday to call an apiarist to remove the bees — for a hefty price, I might add. I have a better idea." I cringe beneath the covers.

The queen left with her minions. I *finally* settle down for my nap and wonder which was worse: having bees in my chimney or thinking their buzzing in my ears was a normal part of Cancerland. "Whooo are Yooou?" I repeat to Baby who answers, "Purrfect, purrrfect."

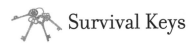 ## Survival Keys

* Celebrate Friendship. True friends can be new, old, or fur. A fair-weather friend is like your shadow—by your side during sunny times but gone when clouds appear.

* Allow friendships to be tested. Dark clouds can be divining rods that will test relationships for you. Use them.

✳ Welcome new friends. A true friend is not
necessarily someone you've know all your life. It's
someone who's with you through the hard times
in your life. They are there with you in the dark,
surrounded by annoyances while also suffering from
trauma and fatigue.

✳ Don't be disappointed. Shadow people are a part of
life; don't depend on them to stand up to the dark,
and they won't let you down.

✳ Expect to lose friends. It hurts when a friend
disappears. But, in the words of Alfred, Lord
Tennyson, "'Tis better to have loved and lost than
never to have loved at all."

Chapter 30

Voices and Stress

But a lifetime of happiness! No man alive could bear it:
it would be hell on earth.
— George Bernard Shaw (1856–1950)

♥ *Affirmation:* I see myself taking correct actions.

I don't stand in the long line at the food-court juice bar. I just walk up and the man behind the counter hands me the drink. My daily Big Dig, named after Boston's restoration Big Dig, is a concoction of juiced fruits, vegetables, and wheat grass.

"I've got them trained," I whisper in response to the surprised look on Jill's and Peter's faces. "The minute they see me walk through the door, they start the drink so I won't be late for my treatment. They're so sweet." What a great way to start off the halfway point of my treatment.

Jill will drive in with me every day until she leaves in a couple of weeks. After treatment, we're going to Chinatown for a meal of dim sum, small steamed dumplings served in bamboo or metal steamers. I haven't been this excited about food in a long time. It feels good to be *pleasantly* excited about something again that isn't crisis related.

Everyone is on time for radiation, so Jill and I zip in and out with the cursory "Hi and see ya tomorrows." It's just as well. Today I'd rather eat than talk. I want to forget about treatment and pretend that I'm back in my old healthy life, if only for a day.

"Has any one seen Carol"? I ask the group the following week. "I didn't see her yesterday or Friday." We're concerned because Carol had complained about the chemo port in her chest being infected, which

170

happens if it's not flushed thoroughly or often enough. These infections aren't surprising if you take into consideration our lowered immune systems.

"It's not only her port that's causing the delay," Harriet answers. "I got worried and called her home. It seems she had shingles during chemotherapy and was given medication that reacted to the radiation. Her doctor has stopped her treatment until she feels better."

I'm stunned. The look on my face must have relayed my feelings to the group.

"Are you okay?" Harriet asks. "Carol will be fine, and I'll keep in touch with her by phone."

I nod. *That could have been me!* If I had told the doctors about my shingles outbreak in the hospital, would I have had the same negative reaction? My guides and my kombucha tea working together saved me again. I say a silent thank-you as I sit down, keeping my thoughts to myself. As much as we share in our little group, I'm not ready to share my spiritual guides. I need this group. Like being gay, there's a bit of the "don't ask, don't tell" policy that goes with being intuitive, so I'm perfectly content to stay in the closet.

Laura, my nurse, says, "Don't get dressed after your treatment, because the doctor wants to see you."

I feel the room spin as my anxiety increases. "You'll see the doctor every Tuesday, so have a seat back in the waiting room. Are you having any side effects?" she asks and sits beside me with folded hands, like the perfect listener. I wonder if anxiety attacks count.

Whenever my routine is altered, I still frighten and immediately prepare for the worst. When life throws things at me randomly, routine seems especially important. It gives order to my chaos. If chaos is reorganization, I won't have a hair out of place — once it grows back.

The nurse leads to examining room number *two*. Synchronicity at work? Do I dare view this as a good omen?

This is the first time I've seen Dr. Harold since my radiation mapping at Brigham and Women's, yet he feels like an old friend.

"You're doing great!" he says as I put my robe back on. "I'll see you next Tuesday."

On the way out from the inner waiting room, Jill laughs. "I thought you weren't going to make friends with anyone during treatment. You guys seem like an old knitting group in there, chatting away and watching out for each other."

So much for my "don't get friendly" rule.

"Some women in the group are burned through to their backs. Is that going to happen to me?" I ask Dr. Harold at my next Tuesday checkup. My nonchalant voice belies my anxiety.

"No. That's why I did an ultrasound before you started your treatment. Remember?"

So, those burned women are not his patients. Maybe the doctors need a little knitting group of their own. Obviously, not all doctors are the same and neither are their techniques. This reminds me of a joke a tennis friend shared over lunch.

Question: What do you call a medical student who graduates at the very bottom of his class?

Answer: DOCTOR!

"Everyone knows stress is a killer," Linda from Cape Cod says. But since my divorce I don't really have stress. And all the other people who used to bother me are dead. So why do I have cancer?"

We sit in shocked silence at her honesty. Our little room is overflowing because the technicians are delayed. Becky is the first to recover and replies, "I don't think that's quite what we meant when we said most people who have a serious illness usually had a prior trauma. You probably had a lot of stress before you got rid of your husband and annoying friends. You've only been divorced a few years, right?" Linda nods in agreement. Becky continues, "We don't get cancer overnight. It takes years to grow from a microscopic cell to something that's visible on a mammogram or can be felt …."

Thus began our Friday discussion on "killer crisis and cancer." We examined how women are accustomed to being the caregivers in relationships, yet often don't know how to say, "Hey, I need a nurturing back rub." After a long day at work they get dinner ready, clean up the kitchen, and see to the kids' homework while doing laundry so everyone has clean underwear. Being a breadwinner, cook, tutor, and maid is exhausting. Women are getting burned out.

So what's my excuse? I have a wonderful husband who quit work to stay home and care for me. I don't work, and I have a housekeeper, but when I look further back, I remember I was under tremendous stress. And the shock is that much of it was of my own making.

If stress played a part in my illness, what could I have done differently to change my outcome? This was the first time I had the emotional strength to look back, rip the bandage off the wound cleaned during therapy with my Wolf/Indian therapist, and examine its progress. I had allowed trauma to affect me by giving up my personal power, and tried to control everything and "make it all better" — the true sign of a caregiver. I remembered a dream I'd had years ago in which I asked my guide why I always felt so lucky and blessed. "It's only a matter of perception," he replied. "Others who see only sadness perceive life as such."

So it all boiled down to one man's gift is another man's baggage. I decided right then and there, in my little knitting group, to distinguish between the things that were my baggage and those that were other people's baggage and not carry or accept their crap as gifts. It was not only unhealthy for me but also counterproductive for them. It's their stuff, so let them choose to carry it or put it down. Next time I feel stressed I'll ask myself: *Is this my shit or theirs?*

Marriage and relationships are often built on roles so people can meet each other's needs. A woman who gives unconditionally might be surprised to discover that her partner is incapable of nurturing. She becomes an "abandoned spouse" when he finds someone else to "meet his needs." Remember: an empty well cannot give water. Taking care of you first isn't selfish, it's smart.

Saturday night, our doctor friend, Cindy, stayed with us. After she gave me a Reiki boost, we talked about the importance of using our intuitive gifts to help others and give back to the universe. "I really want to work with coma patients and see if I can contact them or help them in any way while they're comatose," I told her. Well, today Cindy called from Boston Hospital to tell me she had a little girl for me to work on.

"Her name is Kristin and —"

"No! Don't give me any more information, because it might influence me. I'll tell you what I see. That way you can tell me if I have the right person," I told Cindy. Then I hung up and immediately phoned Patricia with my new idea. "So, I want to see if I can enter your dreams tonight, without waking you, and hand you something. Then, when I talk to you tomorrow, tell me what I gave you, okay? Does this make you nervous?" I asked.

"No, dear," Patricia said. "I think it's a great idea. In fact, I think you should call my friend Penny, who you haven't met, and do the same thing with her."

Distant relatives, Penny and Patricia have also been friends for almost thirty years. Although I had heard about what a great spiritualist Penny was, I hadn't yet had the pleasure of making her acquaintance. This would be a heck of an introduction. Patricia explained, "You and I already have a connection, but you don't really have one with Penny, so it would almost be a blind study. Is there anyone else you could try this on besides Penny?"

"No!" *No one else is going to let me tromp around in her dreams. My few friends would probably consider this idea a nightmare.* "Would you ask Penny if she's okay with this? If she is, then I'll call her." I'd love to have been a fly on that wall.

In 1971 President Nixon declared war on cancer. Forty years later the disease has increased by 50 percent. Have we lost the war? If so, why? Perhaps the answer lies in these words of the ancient Greek physician Hippocrates: "Let thy food be a drug." New research confirms the power of vitamins in food for health. God heals His creations with His creations. The answers often grow right alongside the questions.

What counteracts poison ivy? Jewelweed, the yellow wildflower that grows beside it. What is cancer's yellow flower? Does it, too, grow right under our noses? We can walk on the moon — is curing cancer so much more difficult? What's wrong with that picture?

Back at the hospital support group, our discussion shifted to chemo brain, side effects, symptoms, sex, and tips for survival. By the time we were done with our stories, the nurses came to see what the howling ruckus was about.

"So, as I drove out of the supermarket parking lot," Becky said, "I saw all these people waving at me, so, being friendly, I waved back. I was singing with the radio when I glanced in my rearview mirror. People were chasing me and still waving." We listened spellbound.

"Didn't you notice your groceries were missing?" someone asked.

"Not till I saw vegetables rolling down the street. I just backed up and thanked everyone while they put the ripped bags in the back seat." We roared with laughter because this could have happened to any one of us. "I'm beyond being embarrassed anymore," Becky continued. "If it hadn't taken me so long to find the car keys, I wouldn't have put the groceries on the roof of the car in the first place."

"Am I the only one having tremendous gas?" Cindy asked nonchalantly as she brushed a piece of wig out of her eye. "It's so bad some days I'm afraid to leave the house. I'm constantly farting and apologizing to my family."

"You apologize after you fart?" Becky asked in disbelief. "You are *waaay* too polite. I've been experiencing parting or fissing, depending on how you look at it."

"What the heck is that?"

"That's when you fart and wet your pants," Becky answered.

I laughed so hard I almost wet my pants. But it's true! We're experiencing things that don't even have names, so we make them up to act as descriptors.

"One of the side effects of radiation is bloating, so of course we're going to have gas," one of the girls said. "It's like we're cooking from the inside out. Just think of a fart as a burp from behind." We can make each other feel better no matter how outrageous our problem.

"What about sex? Has anyone else had difficulty with sex?" a new girl asked the group. She's so new we don't know her name yet, but with that question, she's definitely a "keeper." Sex is always a great topic of conversation. By the time we leave, we all have notes scribbled on whatever paper was available. Even the nurses take notes, and we'll stay extra late on sex-talk days because for some of us, that's what sex has become — all talk. We take turns giving advice.

On the way home, we stop in the quaint seaside town of Hull for a gourmet meal at my favorite restaurant, which features panoramic views of the beach on which it is built. Today's treatment was my three-quarters completion point. As I sip my wine, stress melts away, appetite returns, and my mind wanders to Provincetown and the sex shop that helped my marriage during crisis.

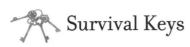 Survival Keys

✳ Don't take a trauma personally. It's an equal-opportunity condition that doesn't discriminate against gender, class, color, or creed. Don't take it personally, and you'll get over it more quickly.

✳ Learn from it. Trauma is also a matter of perception. You can see it as a bad situation or as a learning situation.

✳ Face denial. The earlier any disease is caught the better the chances of survival, and the sooner a crisis is recognized the quicker it can be solved. Denial is often a culprit.

✳ Trust inner guidance. It may trump technology. Technology needs to catch up. The techniques used today to detect cancer are better than nothing, but just barely. Younger women with dense breasts have a 20 percent chance of having their breast cancer missed. Use your inner guidance.

✳ Share sexy ideas. We all want to live and be loved. Sex makes the world go round, yet sex during therapy can be a problem. Sharing sexy ideas can solve problems.

Chapter 31
SEX, DRUGS, AND ROCK 'N' ROLL

Love is a fire that burns longest when sparked
in the heat of passion and stoked with kindness.
— Kathleen O'Keefe-Kanavos

♥ *Affirmation:* I have a wonderful partner, and we are both happy and at peace.

Have you ever wondered *will sex ever be enjoyable again during or after my treatment or trauma?* Your answer may be found in the following pharmaceutical, holistic, and yoga practices. After experiencing painful sex, the fear of intercourse can become a self-fulfilling prophecy. It takes courage to explore an area that has been taboo in our culture for so long — the act and art of lovemaking.

Sex may be 90 percent mental, but the 10 percent that's physical can often be painfully difficult during stress, menopause, treatments, or when vaginal tissues become dehydrated and lose their elasticity. Things don't slip 'n' slide the way they once did. There may also be a loss of libido due to the estrogen-eating chemicals necessary to defeat hormone-receptive cancer, crisis-induced fatigue, and self-image issues.

Hormones stimulate sex, as do healthy energy levels accompanied by a feeling of physical pride. It's difficult to feel sexy with little or no hair, minimally brushed teeth, exhaustion, missing body parts, and all the other unattractive things that may accompany therapy, but by addressing these issues and adopting some helpful hints, you will feel sexy again.

Our sexuality is a big part of who we are. As our bodies change from trauma, illness, and treatment, physiological changes occur that can alter the way we feel about and respond to sex. During the best of times, men and women relate differently to sex. As one book so aptly noted, men are from Mars and women are from Venus. During treatment, we can appear to be from different universes. In her book *The Sexy Years*, Susanne Somers describes the "seven dwarfs of menopause" as Itchy, Bitchy, Sweaty, Sleepy, Bloated, Forgetful, and All-Dried-Up. Yeah, I've met them!

When I explained my sexual difficulty to my gynecologist, he prescribed a vaginal pill called Vagi-fem, an organ-specific hormone therapy. Since my tumor was HR+ (estrogen hormone receptive), I called my oncologist to verify that it would not interfere with my treatment or cause serious problems later. Some hormones can stimulate hormone-receptive cancers.

"Oh," the oncology nurse said over the phone, "my sister is using Vagi-fem because she said having sex while on chemotherapy is impossible for her, too. And a friend is taking it for menopause issues. I'm sure you can take it, but I'll give the doctor your message."

Everyone seems to know someone with cancer. Well, that gives me more people to learn from, just like now. Although I believe the nurse, I want to hear this from my oncologist. He confirms that Vagi-fem is safe to take, so I insert the tiny pill vaginally once a day for two weeks, and then one pill twice a week, and hope I'll no longer hear the songs *Like a Virgin* and *Feels Like the First Time* playing in my head during sex.

The ESTRING°, another answer, is a flexible plastic ring that fits around the cervix and gradually releases low doses of estrogen into the vagina to re-thicken vaginal walls and increase lubrication. It's replaced every three months. "Makes things slip and slide again," a girlfriend going through menopause joyfully announced during lunch.

Another helpful hint came from the wife of a basketball player. Many basketball players have big hands, feet, and...extremities. The petite wife was asked how she handled sex with her husband's large extremity. (You'd be amazed at what women discuss at lunch — and it's not ironing, diapers, or recipes.) "Lubricate and inebriate," was her answer. "A drink of wine and a drop of grease can make all the difference in the world."

I took her advice, but found that K-Y Jelly simply didn't do the job — too sticky. I needed professional help. I drove to a sex shop in Provincetown, Cape Cod's little San Francisco.

The shop I had in mind was on the main street of "P-Town," next to Spank the Monkey, a store with a life-size wall painting of a man spanking the bare bottom of a large hairy monkey. An electric scooter bearing a six-foot-four drag queen dressed as Cher in sequined mini, fishnet stockings, and three-inch spike heels speeds past, sending tourists sprinting for safety right into the claws of a six-foot dancing lobster passing out flyers for the evening's transvestite review. It's a typical summer's day in P-town — positively gorgeous and never boring.

I grab Peter, my emotional support, and head for the door of the sex shop. Once inside, I lower my head to hide my flushed face and rush down the narrow aisles that display leather clothing and whips. I follow signs pointing to the second floor's XXX shop, and pray that I'll immediately find what I need, pay for it, and leave.

Fortunately, the second floor is so crowded that no one takes notice of us. Two middle-aged women huddled with a salesgirl hold packaged electric sex toys and question the contraptions' performance as though they're comparing electric eggbeaters. One woman unabashedly asks which one performs better on what speed. The sight of my gaping mouth interrupts her, and she stops talking and smiles at me. I scurry past them and right into a display of lubricants, knocking bottles and jars to the floor. *So much for being invisible,* I think. To my horror, people in the isles stare as I kneel to retrieve a long, flesh-colored, phallic-shaped bottle as it bounces on its head. Then I grab at the smaller pastel-colored versions that dance around the floor like sugarplum fairies. *Oh, God, help me!*

"May I help you?"

I peer up, arms overflowing with provocative captured containers. I'm alone, sans Peter, and face to face with a grinning salesgirl. *Thank you, God — it's a woman!*

"Well, you see, I have this problem and I didn't know where else to go for help," I stammer in a choked whisper and proceed to let it all tumble out. The only thing missing is the couch and Dr. Freud. I can't believe I'm telling this stranger my most personal thoughts, challenges, and emotions pertaining to sex. To my surprise, she's not only a great listener but spends the next fifteen minutes educating me on the finer points of lubrication.

"Different lubricants fill different needs. Do you want waterproof, long-lasting, water-soluble, or flavored?" *Is this a trick question?* My vapid look says that this is over my head.

"Okay. K-Y Jelly is condom-safe, but tends to get sticky and isn't long-lasting, so you have to reapply it during intercourse if you're going to take awhile. The best lubricants are made in Germany," she continues, reaching for the small, black, phallic-shaped bottle in my arms. *Leave it to the Germans to keep engines running smoother and longer,* I think. "Body Action Xtreme stays slippery for quite some time, even underwater, and it won't interfere with condoms."

"Interfere with condoms?" I repeat. I recall Dr. Barkley advising me to use condoms while on chemo because of the possibility of getting pregnant. I wonder how many baby boomers were conceived with incompatible lubricants.

"Yes. A non-latex-compatible lubricant will dissolve condoms." *There's a lovely thought! What would it do to my insides?* "But this gel," she says, "is compatible and really lasts because it's silicone-based, not water-based. And some lubricants are flavored, but again, those are usually water-soluble. Also, there's the warming formula that heats up with friction," she says, pointing to another suggestively skinny bottle in my hand.

That's the last thing in the world I need! With such a tight space to work in, things tend to heat up naturally from friction without any extra help. I don't want to burn down the bedroom — I just want to have normal sex again.

"The bottom line is that you're going to get what you pay for," she says, and helps me replace the bottles in their shelves, starting with the one that heats up. "Unless they have flavoring, which adds to the

price, water-based products are cheaper than the better silicone for-
mulas, but the best way to tell is to feel the difference," she whispers,
leaning toward me with a sly smile as she opens a bottle. *Oh, shit!
What's she gonna do?* Gently taking my hand, she pours a drop of the
water-based product on the front of it and a drop of the silicon-based
on the back, and then proceeds to rub them briskly. "There, now, feel
the difference?"

There *was* a difference! The silicon was smooth as silk. I looked
around to show Peter, but he was nowhere in sight. "You don't know
how much you've helped me. I was so nervous, but you've truly made
me feel comfortable. Thank you."

"Oh, no problem," she answers, and is instantly joined by another
woman who had been listening from a safe distance. "We take care
of the women and let the men take care of the men. If I can ever be
of further assistance, just ask for me," she says and hands me her card.

*That was so easy, I think. Maybe I should ask about an "eggbeater."
After all, I shouldn't be the only one here without one. I wonder if they
come with one of those little warranty cards you fill out and send in the
mail just in case....*

When I head for the stairs with my little bag of goodies, Peter
miraculously appears from behind a bookshelf containing XXX
DVDs. "So? What did you get?"

"Oh, just the very best lubricant, which, by the way, is made by the
Germans. And a toy."

"A toy? What kind of toy?" He reaches for the bag in my hand.

"I'll show you when we get home. Now that we've got some good
'engine oil,' let's find a great rock 'n' roll CD for later tonight...."

*Wow! Wait till I tell the radiation group about this. Even the doctors
will take notes.*

Yoga practices and meditation are another method of dealing with
sexual challenges. These practices bring your full awareness into your
body, breath, movement, and voice. One such practice is tantra yoga,
which teaches the acceptance of all parts of ourselves and connects
sex with spirit.

After exploring these avenues of enjoyable sex, I've chosen yoga, meditation, and lubrication. I discontinued the Vagi-fems because my concern about hormones negatively affected my state of mind, and a positive mindset is another important part of lovemaking. I've found, however, that the ultimate aphrodisiac is having a good-looking hunk next to me in bed who thinks I'm still desirable and wants to love me till the cows come home. I call that hunk Peter, my significant other, husband, best friend, and lover.

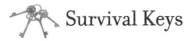 ## Survival Keys

* Laugh. Laughter is medicine.

* Be happy. Happiness is therapy.

* Have sex. Sex makes the world go round.

* Take control of your healing with happiness.

Chapter 32

SWEET DREAMS

If you can imagine it, you can create it.
If you can dream it, you can become it.
— William Arthur Ward (1921–1994)

♥ *Affirmation:* I envision the future I DO want.

It's nearly noon on a sunny Saturday when I roll out of bed and putter around the kitchen making coffee, the phone sandwiched between my ear and shoulder.

"Hi, Patricia. It's Kathy. I hope I'm not keeping you from your nap."

"Oh, hi, dear. No, I'm still up. I saw you in my dreams last night — you walked into the study and handed me a book."

"Yes," I say, surprised to have immediate validation of my dream without even telling her why I was calling. "I thought I'd walked into your bedroom rather than your study, because the study looked very different in your dream from the one we usually sit in. There was a work desk in it."

"Right, well, that's my upstairs study, where I do all my writing. I converted one of the bedrooms last year. You've never been up there, but that's where I was sitting in my dream."

Well, I've been there now, I think. *Nice study.*

My next call is to Penny, with whom I'd never spoken. I feel awkward. How do you tactfully ask a stranger if she saw you in her dreams? It sounds like a bad pickup line at a bar, right along with "If I tell you I love your dress, will you hold it against me?"

"Hi, Penny. We've never met, but I've heard so much about you

184

from Patricia that I feel like we're old friends. Is this a good time for you to talk or should I call back later."

"This is an excellent time, and I know who you are and why you're calling."

Is that a good or bad thing? I wonder.

"I saw you in my dream last night," Penny says, "and though I'd never met you, I knew it was you. You handed me a rose in my garden. How did you know I love flowers?"

"I didn't." I answer honestly. "I just asked my guides to please take me to you if I had permission to do this work with coma patients, and to give you something we would both remember. I ended up beside a house with a beautiful flower garden. A rose was in my hand, and you were sitting on a gardening stool."

"Yes, you handed me the rose, didn't say a word, and then you were gone. The flower garden you're describing is on my property on Nantucket Island. That's where I am right now. My house on the Cape doesn't have roses."

I really did it! I think after I hang up. I guess I have permission to do this work, so now I'll try this with little Kristin. But how will I know if I'm successful? I can't call Kristin and ask if she saw me in her dream. She's in a coma and can't speak.

A voice in my mind answers my question with a single word: *Believe.*

I've started my fourth week of radiation. After the treatment, I have an appointment with Dr. Barkley for my monthly checkup. Another full day of doctors and tests.

"What side effects are you having?" His smile matches his bowtie as he sits on his little black stool.

"You mean other than a sunburned breast and fatigue?"

Dr. Barkley peers over his glasses to see if I'm serious. "Not from radiation. From Tamoxifen."

"Oh. I don't think I'm having any side effects from it. I feel fine. Sometimes I feel like I'm getting ready to menstruate or ovulate, but nothing happens."

"When was your last menstruation?" Dr. Barkley asks.

I didn't even have to refer to my two-year pocket calendar, always in my possession. Today is one week shy of six months since my very last period, on the first day of chemo. How could I forget! Chemo and menopause all wrapped up in IV bags of shit and giggles.

"Good. Let's get a blood test and I'll see you in a month."

I ask Deana, my chemo IV nurse, to draw my blood. After all, we both know the drill, and to be brutally honest, I don't think anyone else wants me. As my crimson fluid fills the tube, I can't help but wonder what they're looking for in these blood tests. On second thought, I don't want to know. I'm afraid I'll turn into a hypochondriac and have symptoms of something I don't have when I didn't have symptoms for something I did have.

Don't dwell on the past, I tell myself as Deana replaces the needle with a Band-Aid and folds my arm to keep the vein from bruising. Anyhow, I've decided that Saturday night, while nestled comfortably in bed, my bra filled with RadiaDres hydrogel sheets, I'll see if I can contact little Kristin during a meditation. I don't know what to expect since I've never entered anyone's coma. Could I possibly get stuck there? How will I know if I am? *Shit!* I make a mental note to ask my guides to safely take me to Kristin *and* return me.

"Hi, Kathy, this is Penny." The calm voice on my answering machine belies its true level of anxiety. "If you get a minute I'd really like to speak with you. It's rather urgent." I've just gotten home from my midweek Boston drive and am feeling tired, but I remember how open Penny had been, allowing me into her dream. I return her call immediately.

"…So, you see," Penny explains calmly, "I have to make a choice, and with the doctors not even sure if it is cancer, I don't know whether to go to the one in Boston who wants to perform a complete hysterectomy or the woman here on the Cape who only wants to remove the ovary with the suspicious area on it. I hoped you could speak with the guides and see what they have to say about all this. And please ask them if the spot is cancerous."

I was having a panic attack just listening to her — for her. "Patricia and I were so impressed with how helpful and accurate the spirit guides were when Tom went through his surgeries. I hope they'll talk to you about me."

"Of course I'll try to contact your guides," I said. "I'll call you as soon as I know something." I cover my face with my hands. How could she say all that so calmly? I would have been in tears if not in hysterics. The "C," word — Cancer — still scares the hell out of me — even when it isn't mine.

I sit in our sunroom, quiet my body and mind, and immediately go to my special place, accessible only by astral travel. It looks like a Greek temple without walls, surrounded by five Greek columns. It's incredibly peaceful, and it's here that I often converse with my guides when I'm not in a nightly dream state. I'm in a meditative state, different from my pop-up dreams. When I come here, I know where I am because this is my place. When my guides take me through a pop-up, I have no idea where we're going until I get there.

"Why do you want us to give you information that will be confirmed by tests?" the guides ask. "We do not do hoops and neither do you."

Well, that was direct. I explain that I'm unsure of my medical readings, but if I could give one that could be verified by medical tests it would boost my intuitive confidence.

After a long pause, the single word "Okay" is quietly uttered.

"Yes, the spot is cancerous, but it doesn't matter whether she removes just the ovary or her uterus and both ovaries, because only that one ovary is affected. It won't make any difference if everything is removed or left intact," the grinning guide says to me. He is an ancient Asian dressed in colorful red-and-white flowing silk robes, and has long, white braided hair and a white beard. I had watched him walk up to my platform on a cloud pathway. I was pretty sure he was not one of my guides because my guides look like Franciscan monks or Druids with brown hooded robes, knotted rope belts, and sandals. I seldom saw my guide's faces because they kept their hoods up.

"Oh, yes. That was Ning. I've been feeling him around me," Penny says when I describe the Asian and tell Penny what he said. Her guide has a name; mine has a hood — different people, different guides.

"Well, I've decided to go with the local woman who wants to take just the one ovary because she doesn't think there's cancer involved, just a cyst. The operation is set for Friday. Let's keep our fingers crossed. At the time of the procedure, Patricia is going to light a candle for me and tend to the flame." Patricia always does this for people going through surgery. "You'll be having radiation right at the time of my surgery," Penny says.

"I'll put you in my radiation meditation." The words are out of my mouth before I have time to realize I might have frightened her with the thought of radiation beams and her surgery in the same healing bubble.

"That will be wonderful. Thank you," she says.

 ## Survival Keys

* Tune in to your guides. Everyone really does have guides.

* Know that you are their job and they take their job seriously.

* Be aware of your dreams. They are an important link to your guides.

Chapter 33

BECKY'S MELTDOWN

No! just means start again — at the next higher level.
— Kathleen O'Keefe-Kanavos

♥ *Affirmation:* I have keen insight and intuition.

Becky and I show up for our treatment today with matching Fourth of July vests. Brilliant minds think alike. We tell people all the time that we're fraternal twins connected at the heart. Independence Day isn't till Sunday, but it's close enough for us to do our favorite thing — celebrate. I don't think there's anywhere else in the country that celebrates the Fourth like Boston. Flags are everywhere: in windows, on lawns, tied to car antennas and front grills, and all the bars are rocking with people clad in red, white, and blue. I use to think the Fourth of July celebrations on the military bases in Europe were incredible, but Boston has them beat.

Someone from an earlier group had completed her treatment and left a box of chocolates as a parting gift. I avoid candy for weight and health reasons, but seeing the luscious pieces smiling up at me from their individual little paper beds is more than my inner children can stand. They begin to sing a song with the Bo Diddley beat: "*We want Candy!*"

But you know we aren't eating sugar now, I rationalize, hoping to quiet the beat rocking my brain.

"*We know a girl who's tough but sweet / We want Candy!*"

We might not be able to eat just one piece, I counter. Where are my inner adults and inner physician when I need them? They'll get those kids to stop. Without missing a beat, my parents sing, "*Candy's just*

189

what the doctor ordered!" I munch on the delicious chocolate and prepare to leave for the weekend. Fridays are big days because we gaze back on a week of completion and forward to one of challenges. Is that light at the end of the tunnel growing a little brighter? So close, yet still so far away.

Saturday morning I meditate to contact Kristin in her comatose state. I say a short prayer of thanksgiving and ask to please be taken safely to and from Kristin. By the time I finish this part of the meditation, I've reached my special place floating high in the sky with pathways for travel between realms of realities and time known as the time continuum.

I take my guide's hand (the first time he has offered me his hand) and find myself in a hospital room looking down on a little girl I don't know. She lies on a bed and is hooked up to IV tubes and monitors. The sounds of life support fill the room. The child, who is very small and frail, appears to be three or four years old. Her pale skin blends with the white sheets.

"Kristin?" I ask, checking to see if I'm in the right hospital room.

"I'm here," answers a tiny voice from above Kristin's body. I look up at a smiling little girl in a pale yellow dress holding hands with a woman who appeared to be twenty-two years of age.

"My name is Kathy, and I'm here because your doctor asked me to see how you're doing. Who is that holding your hand?"

"Lydia. She's my friend," Kristin replies.

"Why are you out of your body, Kristin?"

"It hurts in there. It's better with Lydia," she says, swinging Lydia's hand in hers.

"Well, why don't you leave with Lydia? Then you won't hurt anymore."

"It would make my family too sad. Mommy would be the saddest. She still cries, so I have to stay here."

"It's time to go," my guide says, reappearing beside me. Before I can object, I'm back in my bedroom finishing my meditation.

I phone my doctor friend, Cindy, the next day to see what I can find out about Kristin's pain and about Lydia. "Happy Fourth of July, Cindy. I was able to see Kristin in her hospital room and wanted to share what I found out." I went into detail.

"That's exactly what Kristin looks like," Cindy says. "She's been having strokes since she was two, and after this last one she has severely limited brain function. That's why she's on life support and *yes*, her mother would be *very* upset if she died. She goes to the hospital daily with family members, especially Kristin's sisters. I have no idea who Lydia is, since I'm not Kristin's primary-care physician. It's interesting that she said her body hurts. I didn't think she was aware of too much because of her brain damage. When I go in to work tomorrow, I'll speak with her physician about that. From what I understand, there's not much hope for Kristin, as she's been in a coma for three months with no change. In fact she seems to be getting worse, but you said you wanted a challenging coma patient, so I gave you Kristin."

"Hi, Kathy, it's Cindy." the voice on the phone greets me. "I hope I'm not calling too late. I want to know how you're doing with your last week of treatment and to tell you that I spoke with Kristin's doctor about her possibly being in pain."

"Did you tell her about my astral travel into Kristin's room?" I ask, a bit shocked at the thought of two conservative Boston doctors having such a radical discussion.

"No," Cindy chuckled. "Though she does know that I do meditation and Reiki with some of my patients. Anyhow, she said she would check into pain medication for Kristin. At this point I don't think anything could hurt because Kristin's not showing signs of improvement. Just thought I'd let you know. It'll be interesting to see if you can contact Kristin again."

We end our conversation with the promise to speak again soon, and while Dr. Cindy prepares for the next patient in her office, I prepare to have another chat with Kristin.

I settle comfortably into bed beside an already sleeping Peter, slip into my meditative state, and ask permission to speak with Kristin. Before completing the request, I'm back in Kristin's hospital room, gazing up at her, still floating above her body with Lydia.

"Hi, Kristin. Do you remember me?" I ask from the foot of her bed. She nods yes as the sounds of life support pull my gaze down to the tiny body beneath the sheet, reminding me of my mission. "Why don't you try getting back into your body? Look at it. It's such a nice body. Maybe now it won't hurt, and if it does, you can get back out." I expected Lydia to either agree or disagree, but she continued to silently float beside Kristin, holding her hand.

"I don' know how to get back in because I don't remember getting out," Kristin replies.

I was stumped. "I remember when I had some teeth pulled out. It really hurt, and the doctor gave me medicine that didn't make the pain go away, it just made me sick." I open my mouth and point to my missing wisdom teeth. "Anyhow, this little boy showed up in my room when I was in pain, just like you are," I point to her body in the bed, " and he asked me if I wanted to get out of my body and fly around for a while. I told him I was afraid of heights and falling, but he told me I couldn't fall if I didn't have a body." Kristin and Lydia laughed. "He showed me how to slide out of my body through my head, and we flew to the beach. Then he brought me back home and showed me how to slide back into my body through my head. My mouth didn't hurt as badly anymore."

"How did you get back in?" Kristin asked.

"He told me to put my feet on my head and think "IN" and I just slid into my body. You can try the same thing." At that moment my guide reappeared, alerting me that my time had run out, so I quickly added, "Just try it with one foot while you hold onto Lydia. If your body still hurts, pull your foot out." Before I could get a yea or nay from Kristin, I was back in my bed in the dark, listening to my husband's rhythmic breathing.

"I'm going to die!" Becky cried into her hands. "I don't know why I'm going through all this treatment. I'm not going to live anyway. This is all a waste of time that I don't have!"

"What? Becky! What's wrong?" I ask, and sit beside her, my arm around her shoulder. This is not the laughing Becky I know. Or is it? The words "laughing on the outside, crying on the inside" came to my mind as I hear her sobs turn into full-blown crying. Treatment fatigue made us all cry easily. That was a group discussion last week, but there had to be more going on here. The new girl that Becky had jokingly told, "You'll know if the radiation treatments are working when your arm falls off," ran to get a nurse. Becky's wails escalated and her speech became barely intelligible.

"All this shit I'm going through is only going to keep me alive for five more years. That's what all the information says. I feel so tired I can't even fix my son his favorite meal when he comes home from college for the weekend, and I'll never see my daughter graduate from college or get married. Why am I doing all this when I'm going to die anyway? I should be home with them, not wasting what little time I have left here!"

I didn't know what to say. I wanted to cry with Becky. Two nurses appeared on either side of her, lift her off the chair, and, with Becky sandwiched between them, rush to an examining room. I stand up to go with her, but the technician says I'll be treated next.

After my treatment, Becky is nowhere to be found. The energy and air had been sucked out of the room with her, and our little group is extremely pensive. The sharing we just experienced has squelched further sharing. The same psychiatrist the chemo nurses had called for me enters Becky's room. She's in good hands: that psychiatrist saved my life and possibly the lives of others around me my first day of chemo. I'll have to wait until tomorrow to see how my friend is doing. I leave for home with a heavy heart.

The next day, before I have a chance to ask what everyone else in our little group was wondering: *What the hell happened, yesterday?* Becky reassures me, "I'm fine, really I am."

I sit beside her in my medical gown, reach over and take her hand to reassure us both. "I just had a little meltdown," Becky says. "I'm allowed to have one once in a lifetime, and I just had mine," she continues with an apologetic grin and a shrug. Her sense of humor reassures us. We're such a close-knit group that if one of us gets cut, the others all bleed.

"Do you think your meltdown was free-floating anxiety?" I ask.

"No. I think it was all the crap I've been reading about my chances of surviving a five-centimeter tumor. Everything says it will be back in five years like clockwork."

"Well, stop reading shit like that, because everyone is an individual, and science equations can't account for the tenacity of human nature," I reply. Next I tell her about the "only happy endings rule," followed by lots of happy endings: the woman on Cape Cod who had the huge tumor removed from her abdomen and demanded that the chemo be put directly into the incision at the time of surgery. She had beaten the odds and now traveled the country telling her story. I also told her about the woman my Cape vein angel told me about during my weekly blood tests. "She had a large tumor and nine lymph nodes affected. She's still alive and goes in for yearly blood tests as part of her checkup routine. There are positive stories out there, and those are the ones we must focus on." Our fellow radiation-group members nod in agreement. They had come in early too, yet I'd been so absorbed with Becky I'd only now noticed them.

"Well, what are we going to talk about today? We're thirty minutes early for our treatments," I say, and launch into my trip to the sex shop in Provincetown. They listen spellbound. "But what if we can't or won't go into a sex shop?" one friend exclaims. I explain that many pharmacies such as Walgreens and CVS carry lubricants other than K-Y Jelly.

"How about food?" another voice behind me says when everyone is done taking sex notes. "I'm a single mom and so tired I can't decide whether to go to McDonald's or Kentucky Fried Chicken. By the time I get off from work and pick the kids up from school, I'm too exhausted to sit in the McDonald's drive-through lane. The other day I actually fell asleep in my car waiting for the food to be handed out the window, and my son woke me up. It's a good thing I had the car in park. KFC is quicker, but I did that last night. Any thoughts?"

"You shouldn't be eating at either of those places," Becky answers. "A regular diet of that crap could kill a horse." Yep, the old Becky was back.

"When you're raising a family alone, working, and going through crisis, you learn early that you must pace yourself and prioritize. After a long workday and treatment, cooking is way down on my list, and I'm on a tight budget until the court forces my ex to pay up," a voice says from over my shoulder. I can tell by the southern drawl that it's Linda from the group before us. She had been changing out of her hospital gown yesterday when Becky had her crying episode, and the emotion of the moment had bonded her to our group. It's amazing how the sight of vulnerability unites and changes group dynamics. Here is Linda, a perfect stranger till then, baring her soul to us. We rally to comfort her — caregivers to the rescue.

It's sad but true. Some of our friends were busy balancing many life-altering emotional and physical catastrophes at the same time: deception, desertion, divorce, single parenting, breadwinning, crisis, treatment — a juggling act of one's heart, mind, body, pocketbook, stopwatch, and stethoscope that could come crashing down without warning from one wrong move or momentary lapse of attention.

"Do you have a slow cooker, blender, or food steamer at home?" I ask. Linda's colorful scarf flutters as she shakes her head. The look in her eyes reminds me of her tight budget. "New Crock Pots are about twenty dollars at K-Mart, but you can find them at thrift shops for less. Call around to the shops. Crock Pots pay for themselves in both time and money. I got my first one at a second-hand store when I was a poor college student."

Thus began what would become daily discussions on menus, meals, and recipes that took fifteen minutes from beginning to end and were easy, affordable, and healthy. It was a challenge we were up to. I was already using my slow cooker. Before leaving in the mornings, I took frozen food from the freezer, threw it into the crock pot, set it on and six to eight hours later, dinner was served and the house smelled wonderful. If I'm too tired to eat at the table (it happens), I put my meal in the blender with some milk or water and blend a perfect soup for dinner or lunch — especially if my mouth sores are bothering me and I don't want to chew. I also turn on my rice cooker in the morning and it's still warm when I get home. It's like having a private cook prepare perfect meals. Last night I climbed into bed at 6:30, drank my dinner, and fell asleep by 7:30 while watching TV. Pamper yourself! Remember: "I am #1!"

We all agree that the most important meal during any trauma is a breakfast that provides energy to tackle daily challenges. I share my Overnight Oatmeal recipe, cooked in the slow cooker for a hot healthy breakfast that can be stored in the refrigerator up to three days.

Overnight Oatmeal

Prep time 2 minutes; cleanup 1 minute; makes 3 servings

INGREDIENTS:
½ cup steel-cut oats

½ cup 2% milk (or soy milk)

1½ teaspoons brown sugar (you can substitute honey)

¼ cup raisins

½ tablespoon butter

1 teaspoon nutmeg

2 teaspoons cinnamon

2 cups water

⅓ cup ground flaxseed or 1 tablespoon flaxseed oil

DIRECTIONS:
Combine all ingredients in slow cooker and cook on LOW for 8 hours.

NUTRITIONAL FACTS: 1 serving size 265.7g; 287 calories; total fat 9.4g; cholesterol 8mg; sodium 136mg; total carbohydrates 37.3g; dietary fiber 9.8g; sugars 10.9g; protein 16g.

GOOD POINTS = Low cholesterol, low sodium, high dietary fiber.

Survival Keys

✳ Accept life's challenges. Sometimes it takes an experience of major proportions to hurl us out of our habitual patterns.

✳ Focus on today and tomorrow. We can't change yesterday; however, we can use what we've learned to redirect our tomorrow and turn it into a beneficial place for ourselves and for others.

✳ Let crisis be a catalyst. Without the catalyst of crisis we might never find our kindred-soul siblings or fulfill our life purpose.

Chapter 34
VISITORS FROM THE OTHER SIDE

Freedom from Want and Less is More are fraternal twins from the Tree of Life. When you realize you have all that you need and do not want what you do not require, you will be home.
— Kathleen O'Keefe-Kanavos

♥ *Affirmation:* I see clearly both in the physical and subtle worlds.

"So, after Penny's ovary was sent to pathology it was found to be cancerous. She was wheeled back into surgery, and her other ovary and uterus were removed. Pathology said those had no traces of cancer. It was just as her spiritual guide told you. Only the ovary in question was cancerous and nothing else was affected, so it didn't matter if she had a complete hysterectomy or not," Patricia tells me over the phone.

"Anyhow, dear, the reason I'm calling this morning is because Penny has popped a fever and the doctors don't know why. They can't locate an infection. Penny's daughter called to ask if you could speak with Penny's guide to see what's going on."

"Sure. I'll call you back as soon as I know anything."

"Are you sure you're up to this? I don't want you to overtire yourself."

"No problem. I can contact her guides from my comfy bed," I reply and hang up.

Penny's guides were waiting to speak with me. Halfway through my meditation, they showed up and took me to her hospital room where I met people "in spirit" (dead) watching over her. They greeted me as I entered, and all spoke at once. When I left Penny's room I phoned Patricia and told her about "the visitors."

"I just finished speaking with Penny's daughter," Patricia said. "She doesn't know who the people are that you saw in Penny's hospital room, but it turns out that you're right, the infection is in the stitches, and they did use the wrong kind. Apparently they were mislabeled, and the doctor used them on a number of patients who developed infections. Now they have all have to be removed. It's unbelievable what goes on in a hospital, but even more unbelievable is how the guides got that information. Tell me again about the people in the hospital room because Penny said the nurse you described with the short, curly black hair is her nurse. So you were in the right place. You said you saw the living nurse in black and white while the "passed over spirits" in the room were in color?"

I explained again how, midway through my meditation, I found myself in Penny's hospital room rather than at my special place in the sky. Penny was asleep while the room was full of people dressed in colorful clothing conversing with one another. The nurse, however, was in black and white and seemed oblivious to the commotion in the room. I practically astral-traveled on top of her when I entered.

"Hi. Penny has a bad infection in her sutures because they're the wrong kind. They don't dissolve. It's going to take her six months to completely get over this complication. She needs a new doctor, too. I don't like the one she has," an attractive lady in her thirties with shiny shoulder-length brown hair and dressed in 1950s clothing said to me once I reclaimed my composure. "What do you think, dear?" she asked, turning to a handsome gentleman peering down at Penny.

"Yes, I quite agree. But we will stay until she is better, which should be soon."

"Who are you?" I finally managed to ask, surprised by the people, their conversation, and their automatic assumption that I had expected to see them.

"Oh, we're family. I'm Linda, this is my husband, Kevin," she said of the tall dark-haired gentleman who turned and smiled at the mention of his name, "and this is our son Jeff." He appeared to be about seventeen, stood by his mother, and hadn't spoken a word the whole time. At this point they all moved closer together, with Jeff in the middle, and struck a pose. "We're in the family album," she said with a smile just before my guide showed up and whisked me back home to my body and bed.

"What exactly is astral travel and speaking with spirit guides?" a close friend asked me over coffee one day. "I want to understand it but I can't. How do you do what you do when you do it, and how do you control it? Are you always processing information coming in and are you "going out" all the time? How do you not go crazy? You're not intuitive all the time, right?"

"Let me take those questions one at a time. I'll answer your last one first: Yes, I'm always intuitive, even when I'm not meditating. I'm just turned-down, but never off." I looked around the café to make sure we had no eavesdroppers. This conversation was going to get intense as I tried to explain abstract intuitive concepts in concrete terms to a non-psychic.

"I call my kind of processing multitasking on parallel planes, or not-only-but also." Everyone does it automatically, just not to my degree, and some of us do it more than others. Here's how it works. On a day-to-day level, everyone is constantly in the present, thinking about the past and making plans for the future while mentally traveling, without trying or being aware that they're doing it. An example would be chewing gum while watching for traffic when you cross the street and thinking of the great sex you had recently and imagining having it again in the future. You are mentally right there in the past sex act, and tasting your gum while dodging traffic that hasn't reached you yet. This is a form of applied astrophysics that incorporates quantum mechanics and Einstein's general theory of relativity. Sounds complicated, I know, but we do it all the time. Your mind, or memory, doesn't distinguish between past, present, and future because in the time continuum of thought they're all the same. While awake, you daydream, which is a form of meditation. Remember in school when we were told to stop daydreaming, that daydreaming would get us nowhere? Well, daydreaming is how I get everywhere. Controlled daydreams are how I access the door to the past and to people in spirit form, to bring back information for the future. There isn't a past door, present door, or future door. It's one door that goes to one place that contains all three at once."

She continues to stare at me intently, body language open but questioning, both hands tightly clasping her coffee cup. I hope she's still my friend when I'm finished. Hell, I hope *I'm* still my friend when I'm finished. This is some pretty deep stuff, and I've never explained it before. I might scare the hell out of myself before I'm done. I sort through the files in my mind for information concerning this subject from the Psychic Academy and Jeanne's invaluable lessons, which seem to constantly be relevant now.

"Another perfect example would be dreams," I continue with a reassuring smile. Surely this would be a good analogy and one that she could understand from her own experiences. "I don't know how many times I've heard people say to me, "I swear I was really there talking to my deceased friend in my dream." Well, that person probably *was* there, talking to that deceased friend. There are dreams *and then there are dreams*... know what I mean?"

She begins to nod her head in agreement, but then switches the direction to no. "I don't dream," she says.

So much for that analogy, I think, and start again, from a different angle. "You sleep, don't you?"

"Of course."

"Well, then, you dream, too. You dream while you're in the REM level of sleep: Rapid Eye Movement. You know how in movies when the doctor bends over the patient in a coma and sees her eyes moving beneath her eyelids? Well, that patient is in a dream state, participating in the dream. And even in delta and theta sleep, the deepest level and the hardest to remember, you dream. Even a sixteen-week fetus in the womb has REM and dreams.

"Remembering dreams takes practice but it's possible to learn how. It's like any other skill — some people are naturals, and others have to work at it. Leave a notebook and a pen beside your bed, and if you awaken during the night, maybe to go to the bathroom, or when you open your eyes first thing in the morning, write down what you think you remember from your sleep. Answer these simple questions:

1. Do I remember any part of a dream from last night, any animal, person, or place?

2. Do I feel happy or sad right now?

3. What color would I call my sleep?

4. What name would I give my dream, even if I can't remember it?

Don't worry about giving it a wrong color. This isn't a life-and-death situation, and if you give it a wrong color, I'll bet your dream tomorrow night will tell you all about it and will make sure you remember the correct color when you wake up," I say with a laugh. She's not laughing, and I can tell by her serious look this may have been TMI, too much information. "Did that answer your questions?"

"Some of them. But tell me more."

"Okay. Learning to speak with yourself through dreams after being silent for years begins a baby step at a time. When you started school to learn to read and write, one of the first things you learned was your colors and numbers and what they meant. People are not purple and the sky is not red, unless you're psychic and see auras, but I won't go there now. In dreams, however, people and things can be any color, and that's where you're communicating with yourself by using pictures and symbols. You're learning your own dream language. You talk to yourself during the day when presented with a challenge. Some call it sub-vocalizing. If you speak to yourself during the day you can speak to a deeper part of yourself at night. When you communicate in a dream with people you do or don't recognize, that could be astral travel or it could just be a dream, a movie for entertainment."

"Well, how do *you* know the difference?" she asks, looking bewildered. "How do you know the difference between regular versus psychic versus an astral travel dream?

"By validation from people on the earth plane. The people in my astral travel dreams tell me where I am, who they are, and why I'm there. That information is later confirmed or validated by family and friends here on the earth plane when I tell them whom I spoke with and what I saw."

"Does this happen all the time, every day — like is it happening right now?"

I hope my guides are here to help me with some of these questions. I never imagined I'd have this conversation when we sat down for coffee. "Fortunately, I'm able to turn my psychic volume up and down. If I couldn't, I'd probably go crazy, which often happens to people who can't control the flow of information that comes into their minds. It would be like walking around with a TV or radio on your shoulder all the time, day and night.

"How do you turn it up or down?"

"Well, my guides and I have been working together for a while now. When I was two years old I had an imaginary friend named Gee-Gee who shielded, protected, helped, and taught me how to turn my volume up and down. When I was in fifth grade Gee-Gee disappeared, and I think perhaps he became a full-fledged guide for me shortly after that. I've told my guides many times that I can't do this work all the time or I'll burn out or get killed in an accident from the constant distraction, so if they want me to help people, they must agree to keep me safe and act as a filter system or buffer for me. Only that which is of the highest and best from God may come through to me. I won't speak with anything of a lesser vibration, so all the people I've spoken with from both sides have been good people. You see, I'm really nothing more than a telephone line to the other side, and as a telephone line people must get permission to call me and I must get permission to answer or call them. The Law of Permission is one of the highest laws governing both realms. Nothing can be allowed to pass through that thin veil between worlds without permission. I can't just look at someone and say 'I think I'll see what's in store for her in her life today.' First that person must ask me for help. That gives me permission to pick up the phone and see if anyone from her soul grouping or guides on the other side wants to talk. I use my meditation as the telephone. I'm speaking in analogies. I don't actually pick up a phone. You know that, right?"

"Yeah. I think so," she says, still clutching her now cold coffee. She hadn't taken a sip.

"And if they don't want to speak to me, I must respect that and mind my own business, but I've never had that happen. The people on the other side have always been very open, communicative, and polite — more polite than I am. I'm usually too shocked to introduce myself. I'm working on that. But all I need to do is ask and trust that my guides will keep me safe, bring me back, and help me turn down the volume when I'm done."

"Do you always have to be in a meditative state to get information?"

"No. Well, kind of. My meditative state can be so quickly achieved that I can ask a question that's heard on the other side but the answer might not come back for hours, maybe when I'm doing something else, like cooking or reading. Or the answer might come instantly; however, I've asked my guides to not allow information to come through when I'm driving a car or playing tennis, because I don't want to have an accident or get hit in the face with a ball, and they've been very good about it."

"How do you know you have the right person?"

"Again, that's where my guides come in. An intuitive vibrates at a different frequency than regular people, and that vibration attracts spirits like moths to a flame. There are many spirits out there looking for a phone to call home, so when I put a call out or guides bring one in, I trust them to keep unauthorized spirits off my line. Most important, confirmation from living people about the dead is the key to answering your question."

"You're way more than a telephone line. Does this ever scare you?"

"Not anymore. When I was little I used to get scared when I saw and heard ghosts and knew that they saw me watching them. But, again, no one and nothing has ever hurt or even touched me."

"Wow! This is so difficult for me to comprehend. I don't think I have a psychic bone in my body. But you've answered my questions."

"If someone can articulate a question, they're ready for the answer," I say as we prepare to get more coffee, "or you'd have run out of here an hour ago. Instead, you asked and listened with an open heart and mind."

And that was the end of that discussion, for now . . . .

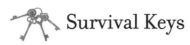 Survival Keys

✳ Pay attention. Daydreams are important and can relay messages and information needed for healing.

✳ Be open. Intuitive gifts may grow stronger during times of crisis.

✳ Be patient. New and old friends may have a lot of questions and confusion around your choosing to follow your guides and higher instincts in the face of crisis.

Chapter 35
THE FINISH LINE AND DEPRESSION

*Our brightest blazes of gladness are
commonly kindled by unexpected sparks.*
— Samuel Johnson (1709–1784)

♥ *Affirmation:* I am safe to be.

"Congratulations! You're almost done, Kathy," Dr. Smith says, looking at my chart. I remember Dr. Smith: he's the new intern who accompanied Dr. Harold during last week's "damage-control" checkup. "I'm seeing Dr. Harold's patients today while he's at a meeting. Are you feeling fatigued? Any aches and pains?"

Is it my imagination, or are these interns getting younger every day? He's at least six foot three, with wavy brown hair, and looks like he's seventeen years old.

"The only soreness I have, besides my red breast, is my collarbone. It seems to hurt right here if I push on it," I explain, placing my index finger on the small spot.

"I've never seen that before, have you?" he asks the nurse. "That's not normal."

Seeing the immediate look of terror on my face, the nurse quickly answers, "I think it's a result of the radiation on her bone, and yes, I've seen it before."

My inner children scream at the top of their lungs: *Oh, please don't let there be a problem. We're so close. No more trains in the tunnel!*

"I'll leave a note for Dr. Harold, and he can take a look at it tomorrow," Dr. Smith concludes and promptly closes my chart in preparation to leave.

"No, you won't!" I hear someone say, and realize it was I. "I won't leave until I see him today, even if it means going over to Brigham and Women's right now and waiting till he can see me." I couldn't believe I was saying this to the doctor. It was like someone had taken over my body — and I was glad they had!

"This is something that can wait until tomorrow," Dr. Smith repeats, so I repeat myself, too, and settle in on the examining table to make my point. He can't simply drop a bomb on me like that and then expect me to quietly and obediently suffer till tomorrow. Right now tomorrow feels like a lifetime away, and I make it perfectly clear that I'm not going to get dressed or leave. Dr. Smith leaves the room.

Five minutes later, Dr. Smith says, "I just called Dr. Harold, and he said he'll come over after his meeting and take a look at you. It may be awhile, so if you want to get dressed and wait where it's more comfortable," he says, pointing to the chairs in the waiting room, visible through the open door, "we'll call you as soon as he arrives." When I didn't move, Dr. Smith left again.

"I'll bet you think I'm a real pain in the ass," I confess to the nurse as she helps me get dressed, "but I don't want to worry all night. If something is wrong, I need to know now."

She chuckles and hands me my belt. "I didn't want to say anything in front of the doctor because he is the doctor," she says in a very low voice, "but this is very normal. I see it all the time, and it *is* from the radiation. But I'm glad Dr. Harold is coming over, because I don't want you to be worried about this. And yes, tomorrow can seem like an eternity. Have a seat in the waiting room, and I'll come get you when Dr. Harold arrives."

"What do you mean something might be wrong and you're waiting for Dr. Harold? What could be wrong?" Peter asks calmly. The terror written all over his face must mirror the terror on mine because he grabs and hugs me. The *look* begins to lessen as I reiterate what the nurse had told me. By reassuring him, I slowly begin to reassure myself and can finally take a deep breath. Unfortunately, I've now learned what the phrase "frozen with fear" means. You can't breathe when you're frozen with fear, and a warm hug can really help.

"Is this the spot that hurts?" Dr. Harold asks two hours later as he presses on the slightly extended bone beneath my collarbone.

I grimace with pain and squeak, "Yes!"

"That's arthritis in the bone from radiation. It's quite common," Dr. Harold says, as much to me as to Dr. Smith, who's standing beside him in the examining room.

"Am I going to have that forever?" I ask as he helps me sit up on the table.

"Probably, but it won't be as sore as it is right now. You're fine, Kathy. You can get dressed now, and I'll see you tomorrow."

What's my final thought on this whole episode as I finish dressing? I hope Dr. Harold chewed Dr. Smith's butt off for frightening the shit out of me like that.

The next morning questioning, fearful faces greet me as I enter the radiation waiting area. You could hear a pin drop and cut the anxiety with a knife. Afraid someone else had broken down I scanned our little group to see who was missing.

"Is everything okay?" Becky asks nonchalantly. It takes me a second to realize that in our tiny, close-knit group word travels at the speed of light; everyone was aware that all had not gone well with my checkup yesterday. They had watched me disappear into a room and not come back out; much like Becky had the day of her crying episode. I had planned to tell them about my "sore spot and the intern." I was simply waiting for a segue. Guess I got one.

"I'm fine. Thanks for asking, but I want to share my ordeal with you so you won't be frightened or caught off guard if it happens to you." Our story for the day was: Defiant Kathy refusing to leave, self-advocating, and demanding, "I want my doctor, now!"

"That jerk!" Becky explodes. "Doesn't he know he shouldn't be speaking in front of patients like that? Doesn't he understand how easily we scare and that he's just an intern?"

"I'll bet good money he does now," I answer with a laugh. "I'll bet he's running around with stuffing in his shorts while he waits for his chewed-off butt to grow back." Everyone, including the nurses, who I was unaware were listening, broke into laughter. (Over time I came to know that the nurses were always listening, always there in the background, out of sight, never intrusive, but always available at a moment's notice. They were the best!) We all heave a sigh of relief as the scary moment passes and humor returns to the group.

"On another note, has anyone else found that when you go shopping now you shop till you drop, buying all kinds of things you don't even want?" Linda from the Cape asks, brushing her Elizabeth Taylor-style black wig back from her face and fixing the group with her lash-less Betty Davis eyes. "I even leave the tags on clothing because I know I'll return it in a couple of days after I recover from my shopping spree. I mean, I can't believe some of the crap I buy. When I get home and take it out of the bag, it's like I don't even remember buying it."

"*Ja*," Anna, a tall German girl with spiked blond hair pipes in. "It's like an alien took over your body and you are shopping like there is no tomorrow." Anna was on vacation in Boston when she found a suspicious lump. She's now undergoing radiation without chemo and is anxious to return home to Germany. It wasn't long before we were giving examples of the crazy stuff we'd been doing and buying, no matter the cost.

What Anna said echoes in my mind: "*We are shopping like there is no tomorrow.*" Is something happening on a subconscious level, deeper than distraction with a credit card that could put us in the poorhouse if we aren't already there? Are we afraid we have limited time or no tomorrow and are therefore trying to acquire all the things we ever wanted in life and may never have the time to possess? Are we living in the moment because we're afraid we only have today, now, this one fleeting second? Are we acting out with credit cards what Becky acted out with tears, and if so, who is being more honest with her form of emotional therapy?

We all stay late and have one of our most important group discussions. The nurses sit with us, drawn by the intensity of our chat group. Some of us were displaying bipolar disorder — a chemical imbalance.

I'm saturated with chemicals right now, clean up to my eyeballs, so I'm not surprised that I'm displaying many of the symptoms. We all discuss our symptoms and find them to be surprisingly similar. The best way to describe it is with the equation chemo/radiation = manic depression, AKA bipolar disorder. Here are some of the symptoms most of us share:

* You feel so hyper that people around you think you're not yourself, and you do things to prove them right. Example: cooking for a small army or cleaning the house at 3:00 a.m.

* Excessive irritability: Snapping answers to questions, shouting at people, starting arguments, or my personal favorite, hanging up the phone on them. It feels like I'm standing outside my body watching in shock as I fly off the handle. "Whooo are yooou?"

* Oscillating between being more talkative and/or speaking faster than usual, speed rapping, or not responding at all.

* Difficulty slowing down a racing mind, especially at night, resulting in being hyper while sleep deprived. Add that to chemo brain and you have an accident waiting to happen. Maybe with chemo brain I'll forget to be bipolar. Now there's a thought!

* Being much more sexually active than usual, or using sex as a means of control even though chemo can make intercourse painful. Maybe we feel we need to get all the sex we can now because there may not be any on the other side. Sex is not a discussion I ever had with anyone on the other side, but I'll bet it would be an interesting investigation!

* Spending out of control. Yeah, we know that one. In fact it started this conversation.

* And the mother of all symptoms: having all of the above all at once.

There are things that can be done to decrease these symptoms. The one that seemed to help me the most was sharing them with my group and realizing that I was not alone and wasn't awful. Also, there are medications to calm the mind at night to aid sleep. Sleep deprivation exacerbates everything. I hope that when the Molotov cocktail of chemicals finally leaves my body most of these symptoms will diminish, and both my credit cards and I will recover.

Our little discussion concludes with this insight: People under extreme stress live for the moment because tomorrow is fleeting. Though we may have very different individual desires, such as finding a new significant other or winning the lottery, we are women first and foremost. We love to shop. We shop, therefore we are!

Peter and I stay in Boston overnight because radiation fatigue has taken its toll on me. All I want to do is sleep after my treatment. When we arrive home the next day there's a message on the answering machine concerning Penny's operation. Worried that something else bad may have happened, I immediately call Patricia.

"Penny's daughter told her aunt about the people you saw in Penny's hospital room, and the aunt recognized their names as deceased cousins of Penny's. The son was developmentally disabled and seldom spoke. But what really amazed her was the photo she found of them in the family album, in the same pose you described, with their names written on the back."

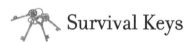 ## Survival Keys

* ✳ Don't lose sight of the fact that there is more to life than what we experience on the earth plane.

* ✳ Anticipate heaven. There's no doubt about it: there is life after death, and loving family to welcome us home.

Chapter 36
ROLLING WITH THE PUNCHES

*To never be challenged while alive is to be already dead. Roll
with life's punches and embrace your challenges.
They are a reassurance of continued life.*
— Kathleen O'Keefe-Kanavos

♥ *Affirmation:* I am open to greater and greater
spiritual awareness.

My perfect Sunday morning is ruined by more cancer woes and another
phone call from hell. The punches never seem to stop coming; it's a
good thing I've learned to roll with them because this one is below
the belt. *As difficult as this is to deal with, Kathy, you cannot physically
afford to get upset at this time. Remember how distraught you were over
your mother. Learn from it. You must truly trust in God and let your father
follow his path in life. Although you are emotionally involved, this is not
your journey, it's your father's,* says the voice in my head as I hold the
phone to my ear and close my eyes.

"The doctor said the shadow on the X-ray in my kidney is suspicious but that it could mean anything or nothing," Dad said as calmly
as possible.

There is another fucking train coming at me, and this time it isn't
even mine.

If it weren't for this phone call from Dad, I'd be out of my mind
with joy. I'm on my last days of treatment. Yet I'm living in good news/
bad news; some kind of a sick balance. Give me just good news for
once! I'm tired of this emotional seesaw. It's like life hands me a rose

212

with one hand and slaps the shit out of me with the other. Keep the fucking flower!

In two days, I AM DONE! Hallelujah, free at last! If I had to do this any longer I would seriously consider renting an apartment in Boston. Besides getting through this week, my other goal was to check in with little Kristin and see if she has "tried her body back on." Wow! That sounds really weird even to me — and I'm involved. I hope no one ever gets my journals and reads them, or they'll come and take me away, ha, ha, he, he, ho, ho, to the funny farm, where life is ..." Isn't that how that song from the late '60s went? But right now I need to find Dad the best kidney surgeon in Boston.

Sitting next to me in the waiting room, Laura, my radiation nurse, says, "Dr. Richard is the Chief of Urology Oncology, Chief of Surgery, and the person Dr. Harold recommends." She hands me Dr. Richard's name and phone number. "When you call, tell his secretary that Dr. Harold recommended him to you. Good luck, and keep us apprised of the situation. This isn't something anyone wants to hear, but this is an especially bad time for you," she says sympathetically, and gives me a big hug. Laura knows what I went through with my mother because it's part of my medical history. Now, I might be going through the same thing with Dad, during a time when I should be overjoyed with treatment completion. There are two lights at the end of the tunnel: one is the exit, and the other is another oncoming train. I have to focus on my light and deal with the train later.

Dr. Richard, who usually has a three-month waiting list to see patients, just happened to have a cancellation and has agreed to see Dad for a consultation one week from today. He even called me at home this evening and asked to have all of Dad's records sent to him ASAP. I feel confident in my decision to put this challenge in God's hands. When there's too much to carry, I realize I must let go and let God. His shoulders are much broader than mine and I think He has already answered my prayers.

✳

"Cindy? It's Kathy Kanavos. Listen, I think Kristin is dead. Have you heard anything?" I ask from my cell phone in the car on the way to my last radiation treatment. Peter listens intently while he drives. He has been aware of and interested in my "Dream Work." The evenness of my voice belies my true concern. I told Peter this morning what happened when I tried to contact Kristin. I didn't want to call Cindy late last night because I know how tired she is after a long day with her patients. Besides, if Kristin is dead there's nothing Cindy can do about it in the middle of the night. There's nothing anyone can do.

"No, I haven't heard anything. What makes you think she's dead?" Cindy replies.

"When I astral traveled into the hospital room, Kristin's bed was made up and empty, so I called out, 'Kristin where are you?' She answered me across time and space, saying, 'I went home.' I asked her what she meant by 'went home' and where Lydia was. She said, 'Lydia is gone, and Tigger is with me. We went home.'"

Cindy says, "I'm in the other building right now, but I'm going to shoot across and see if I can find Kristin's doctor and see what's going on. I'll call you later."

The floor of Nuclear Medicine gets absolutely no phone service. I'm antsy while waiting to finish my radiation so I can run up to the lobby and call Cindy back before I see the doctor for my Tuesday checkup. Becky notices that I'm distracted and that I'm not going to spend any extra time waiting around to chat. As close as we are, I'm not ready to share this part of my life with her or anyone else in the group. I can hear it now: "Stop the radiation on Kathy. It's melted her brain and she thinks she's speaking with spirits. Call the psychiatrist back. She already knows Kathy because she took care of her during chemotherapy." Wouldn't that be a kick in the pants? *Who is Tigger?* I wonder. I never met Tigger in the room with Kristin. Was Tigger another guide?

"Hi, it's Kathy. Got your message. Is Kristin dead?" I ask, barely able to breathe.

"I went to the room and found her bed empty, too, and located her doctor," Cindy says excitedly. "Apparently, Tigger is Kristin's favorite character in *Winnie the Pooh*, which her mom bought for her. Kathy, Kristin's not dead. She came out of her coma and went home."

After we hang up I have to sit down and think about all that for a moment. Why didn't I know that she had gone home? Why didn't I end up in her room at home rather than at the hospital? Of course! I didn't ask the guides to take me to Kristin; I asked them to take me to Kristin's hospital room, so they did. I remember asking Jeanne, the Psychic Academy instructor in Virginia Beach, why some of the answers I got from my guides were confusing or were not the ones I had expected. "Because guides answer literally. They'll only do or answer exactly what you ask of them. If you don't understand the answer, ask again, differently, with more precise information. It's part of The Law of Permission. Guides can't volunteer information."

I found that answer confusing, but here it was in action. As a Special Ed teacher I had learned to write behavioral objectives for my students: precise goals with minimal wordage that could not be misconstrued. (Another life lesson from the past applicable to my present.) I found using behavioral objective-type questions the best way to communicate with my guides for specific information. An example would be asking the guides, "Is my name Kathleen O'Keefe?" They would probably say no. I *am* Kathleen O'Keefe, so are the guides playing games? No. My question wasn't precise enough. Had I stated it in behavioral objective terms such as "In this lifetime and at this moment, is my name, according to me, Kathleen O'Keefe-Kanavos?" the answer would have been yes. Sometimes you must be that specific. I hadn't done that this time with Kristin.

Pondering this before going in to see the doctor, I'm transported back to the beginning of my dream works with Kristin, when I asked myself how in the world I was going to do this work when I wasn't even sure how to start. How was I going to get into the dream state of a coma patient and see what I could do to help her make a choice to live or move on? The answer I heard from my guides then applied now: *Believe*. I had just received verification from Kristin's doctor — someone who didn't even know about my work — that my work was done.

Speaking of done, I'm done! I'M DONE! I began my radiation on a Wednesday and I'm ending treatment on a Wednesday. I've come full circle. It's been six months since my cancer was medically discovered — one hell of a half year.

The radiation boost was easy. It targeted only the incision area where the cancerous tumor was removed, because that's the area where tumors most often return. "You may feel sharp pains, like lightning bolts, in your breast for up to five years from the radiation. That's perfectly normal," the nurse tells me on my last day and then hugs me goodbye. I'm glad for the heads-up on any pain I might have after what I went through with my sore collarbone and the intern.

It was Becky's last day, too. When the technicians come out to get me, Becky takes my hand and tells them, "We want to take our last treatment together. Do you think you can fit us both on the table?" We all have a good laugh. For my farewell treat, I've brought a fruit platter, and Becky baked a cake topped with a pink Happy Face. Thank goodness there's no candy!

"These are for you from all of us," Janet, one of our technicians says, handing Becky and me a Certificate of Completion signed by every nurse, technician, and secretary we had ever come into contact with during our treatment. After hugs and promises to say hi when we come in for our monthly checkups, we walk through those heavy metal doors for what I sincerely believe will be the last time in my life. My nightmare in Cancerland is over, and like Alice in Wonderland, I must now awaken and resume my real life. But how does one pick up the threads of a past life after its fabric has been torn to shreds? Life waits for no one.

After rereading that entry I've asked myself a very important question. Why am I keeping this journal? What do I hope to accomplish by torturing myself with memories that are better forgotten? Could I ever relive this experience with the emotional distance needed to view it professionally like a paleontologist discovering an ancient medical device? Perhaps I should throw these journals away. I lived these diaries, and I have trouble believing and understanding them. Maybe at the end of my five- or ten-year cancer-free checkup, I'll have a bonfire and watch all my fears, trials, and tribulations go up in smoke. Now, that sounds cathartic.

Here's a real kick in the pants: I remembered my doctors' appointments but forgot my anniversary. What does that say about my life right now? On July 31 Peter and I were married for sixteen years, and we forgot about it until now, a week later. We had a good laugh followed by a romantic dinner. If surviving this year doesn't make us feel married, remembering an anniversary is a waste of time.

"Everything looks great, Kathy. When will you be seeing Doctors Barkley and Kritchen?" Dr. Harold asks as I button up my blouse.

"Today at 1:00 and 3:00. It's easier to see everyone on the same day and not drive in from the Cape every two weeks." *Besides, I need some time and space between all of this, I think. I really like you guys, but it's time to wean myself away.*

"Well, I won't need to see you for a month. By the way, the head of the administration department contacted me regarding the letter you sent about your excellent treatment here. It really meant a lot to us to have the head of hospital administration receive a letter like that listing everyone's name and position."

"My pleasure," I answer. "I only told the truth."

"Congratulations on your radiation completion," Dr. Barkley says, smiling up at me from his stool an hour later. "You'll need a yearly pap smear while on Tamoxifen, and a bone-density test because Tamoxifen can cause osteoporosis from lack of calcium and estrogen. I hear you're playing tennis again. Have you had any swelling of your arm?"

"My hand swelled after my first game. I slept with my arm above my head, and it was normal by morning. The fluids found a new route out of my arm."

Dr. Barkley studies my arm and says, "I'm writing you an antibiotic prescription. Carry it with you. If your arm suddenly swells, take them and then call me. Lymphedema can strike years after surgery. Okay, get a blood test. I'll see you in a month. Call if you need me."

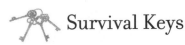 Survival Keys

* Move on. Leaving friends found during times of despair is difficult. Bonds are strong and protective emotions run deep, but a part of the process of life is moving on. It is another rite of passage.

* Pick up the pieces. Soldiers who return from tours of duty in war-torn countries must find and pick up the dropped threads of their previous lives.

* Stay in the flow. Leaving comrades behind is a sweet sorrow, but life does not stand still—it goes on. Stay in its flow or it will pass you by.

Part IV

COMING FULL CIRCLE

Chapter 37

DAD'S KIDNEY CANCER AND TOOTHPICKS

Never abandon life.
There is a way out of everything except death.
— Sir Winston Churchill (1874–1965)

♥ **Affirmation:** I live in the present. I embrace the present and trust that I am exactly where I need to be at this exact moment.

When it comes to cancer in my family, when it rains it pours. At least that's how it has appeared to me these past three years. However, I'm very proud of the way I handled Dad's diagnosis and subsequent surgery for kidney cancer and all the ensuing synchronicities.

It all happened so fast. I guess the person who gazed back at me through the mirror in radiation has completed the metamorphosis, but I'm feeling perturbed by the many tests I've endured without respite. Dad had his cancerous kidney removed yesterday at the same hospital where I had my lumpectomy and Mom had her cancerous colon removed. Surgery didn't help Mom, and I hope I don't have to live through a repeat performance of death. On a positive note, though, it's amazing how people and lessons from my past keep popping up to help me now.

It started with a new secretary who screwed up Dad's appointment with Dr. Richard and suggested that Dad see another doctor. I adamantly refused. I've gotten quite good at digging in my heels. Fortunately, an unexpected turn of events saved the day, when a friend from my

221

chemotherapy floor proved that one can never have too many friends.

"Doreen, what are you doing here?" I ask and give her a big hug. She had heard the ruckus in the hall and came out of her office to see what was wrong. Well, I'm what's wrong. I'm angry with the secretary who messed up Dad's appointment and then tried to hand him off to someone else to save her hide. Doreen, formerly the head nurse from my chemotherapy floor, explains that she was recently transferred to Dr. Richard's floor and is now the head nurse here. Talk about a lucky break — what are the chances of that happening in a lifetime?

"But, what are *you* doing here?" Doreen asks with a look of concern. Everything came spilling out, the whole story of Dad's suspicious shadow, the new secretary, and world-renowned Dr. Richard, whom I had worked so hard to get and had already spoken with on the phone. Doreen puts her finger to my lips and says, "Shhh. Don't worry. This is going to happen." True to her word, two hours later we see Dr. Richard. Then, believe it or not, he had a cancellation for a surgery, so today, one week later, Dad is in recovery, and I'm waiting for the nurses to come out and tell me he's been moved into his room. It's amazing how fast this has all happened, but my life moves at the speed of light right now. I don't dare blink.

"We can't get him to tell us how much pain he's in," the nurse explains as she leads me to Dad's recovery cubicle. Oh, God! I remember this same cubicle when I received my cancer sentence, and that's Mom's right over there. It would have been a bad joke if the real joke had not been two nurses poking Dad with a toothpick. Yes, a sharp toothpick!

"What are you doing and why?" I ask in disbelief as Dad closes his eyes, sets his jaw, and refuses to respond to the nurses' jabs and questions.

"We can't release him to his room until we know his pain level," the nurse answers.

"He's a Green Beret trained not to respond to pain, and since he's still under the influence of anesthesia, he's probably going on his training instinct. Trust me, he's in pain, from the toothpick if not the surgery. Dad?" His eyes fly open above scrunched-up lips. "You're in recovery. The nurses need to adjust your pain medication. Are you in pain?"

He shakes his head no and shuts his eyes — end of conversation.

"Look, he's not in pain, so put that in your charts and send him to his room, because I'm exhausted and I don't want you poking him with any more toothpicks, okay?"

Dad didn't remember any of this when I asked him about it the next day, but he did tell me he wanted to call his girlfriend. And she's only four years older than I. When the hell did *this* happen? Where's that damned toothpick and those nurses when you need them?

Peering over his book at me and the pile of UPS boxes stacked in the middle of the floor, Peter asks, "Kathy, aren't you going to open your Christmas gifts?" This wouldn't be an unusual request except that it's mid-February. Yeah, the party girl is not in the mood for holidays this year. I walk around the boxes on my way to the kitchen for another cup of coffee.

After my therapies were completed and Thanksgiving with Dad *and his girlfriend* was over, we came to our home in Rancho Mirage, California, to spend a quiet Christmas away from colds, flus, and anything else that might remind me of what I went through this past year. The problem is, memories are good travelers, too — no matter where you go, there they are.

Now that I've had time to sit back, breathe, think, and feel, the fact that my mom is really gone and my dad has a girlfriend has hit me. My life is never going to be the same. When, why, and how did all this change happen? My emotions seem to be taking their own course of action. Grief doesn't understand time, space, or place. I want no part of Christmas this year.

"Yeah, Bunny. I'll open them later. I just want to sit here and drink my coffee." Even my inner children aren't interested in the boxes. Things are sad inside my head.

Out of the corner of my eye I see Peter approach with a sharp kitchen knife. Perhaps he has taken pity on me and is coming to put me out of my misery. "Here, I'll cut the boxes open for you. I don't want this pile sitting here at Easter." We plan to spend Easter here. It's important to have things to look forward to, so I'll try to pump myself up for Easter, right after I get over Christmas.

"That's not such a bad idea," I reply. "Maybe we could hide the boxes like big Easter eggs." "*And leave them hidden till next Christmas,*" *my inner grandparents chime in.*

It's one year today since I started my chemotherapy, six months since I finished radiation, and six months since my last journal entry, for a good reason: I've been healthy and haven't had anything to report. No trains have been coming at me. On my birthday, nothing fell out, like my hair, and no voices have contradicted medical reports. Yet I'm depressed.

My bone-density test was at 110% for my age group. I had a Pap smear and gynecological checkup including an ultrasound of my uterus and ovaries as an added precaution since I'm on Tamoxifen. I also had a MRI done on both breasts. I don't trust mammograms, and with good reason. That's exactly what I told the doctors in order to get the MRI prescription. They are not hospital policy. Warning: I now have an attitude and know how to use it! My old radiation group stayed in touch and everyone is doing great. Yet I'm depressed.

One of the biggest compliments I've gotten since returning to "normal life" was from the tennis pro: "Someone has been taking lessons," he said. Little did he know that I hadn't played tennis in seven months and was playing in a full wig. No one I played with knew what I was going through. They assumed I'd been traveling. I didn't tell my tennis team about my health issues for three reasons: (1) I didn't want them to refrain from hitting the ball hard at me, feel sorry for me, or be afraid of hurting me; (2) That unhealthy part of my life is in the past and I want to get on with the future; and (3) I'm a very private person. I didn't even tell Dad about my cancer until I was halfway through chemotherapy, so why would I tell strangers?

I made a new tennis friend in California who recently completed treatment for uterine cancer. It's amazing how people share their cancer treatments like they're discussing pimples.

Ellen explained that after having her uterus and ovaries removed, she'd had to stay in the hospital while liquid radiation, known as brachytherapy, was placed in her abdomen in the "vaginal cuff" of the incision. Although brachytherapy is usually an outpatient procedure, Ellen had to remain hospitalized during this treatment and lie perfectly still. And like my cousin Arty after his radioactive cocktail for thyroid cancer, she was not allowed visitors because she was radioactive. Ellen *did* have visitors, however — visitors from the other side.

Ellen said that her mother and close relatives, all of whom were deceased, came to her hospital room and gave her encouragement by singing to her. The nurses told her husband that she'd been hallucinating when she told him of these visits. (Hearing that brought back memories of the nurses telling me Mom was hallucinating when she saw the man in her hospital room.) Ellen swore it was no hallucination. "What do you think about these visits? Do you think I'm crazy?" she asked. We had a long discussion, which bonded us as friends.

Oh, and Dad's doing well both health-wise and in his relationship with his girlfriend who is also a widow. How do I feel about this girlfriend thing? Well, if Dad is happy then I'm happy. There's evidence that supports the idea that people in a relationship live longer and are healthier than people who are alone. How do I feel about his girlfriend being only four years older than I? More power to him! Makes him quite the stud-muffin. How does Mom feel about all this? I asked her in a dream when I finally recognized her. She looked much younger. "What do you think of Dad's new girlfriend?" She laughed and walked away. *Hmmm.*

"Are you going to marry her?" I ask Dad when his girlfriend comes to stay with us.

It's awkward having this heart-to-heart talk with my father. I remember him asking me similar questions about my dates. "We're both in love," he answers, "but neither of us wants to get married again." I take this with a grain of salt and roll with the punch of watching his girlfriend, instead of Mom, sitting happily beside him at Thanksgiving.

Peter had a more difficult time accepting the two of them sleeping under the same roof, our roof, even though they slept in different bedrooms. I found Peter's distress amusing. "Where have you been for the past twenty minutes?" I ask him. Baby Cakes, our cat, had been talking up a storm. "He's trying to get into the hallway. I have no idea what's wrong with him. Do you?" Peter climbs into bed with a smug look on his face.

"I scattered Baby's squeaky mouse toys all over the hallway floor. If anyone tries to sneak around tonight we'll hear about it," Peter says, snuggling up to me as I peer over my shoulder at him. Yep, the circle of life was complete — we had become our parents' parents.

While in California I had to come to terms with the realization that my hair was coming in curly and *red* rather than straight and blond. I discovered this about three months after finishing my radiation treatments. Yep, I was a redhead with hair as curly as Little Orphan Annie's. I have to say it's a real challenge after having stick-straight blond hair. I always thought curly hair would be easier to care for. Now I'm having second thoughts. All the colors I used to wear — pinks, oranges, and reds — look awful on me. Even the peach fuzz on my face is red. And curly hair takes longer to grow because as it grows it curls.

Here's more synchronicity at work: I began playing tennis again on a USTA team on Cape Cod, and the captain shared her health story with me. I was so impressed that I shared mine with her, resulting in both of us drawing strength and respect from each other. Years earlier, while living in Europe with her husband and children, she had been diagnosed with aggressive adult non-Hodgkin's lymphoma, a malignant cancerous growth in the lymph system. The doctors gave her two weeks to live and sent her home. Not accepting this terminal diagnosis, she returned to the States and underwent chemo and radiation therapy, went into and out of remission for years, and is now disease-free. She beat the odds and surprised everyone. After she came out of her last remission, with no more chemotherapy available, she began meditating and used past-life regression as therapy. Her results were so profound the doctors placed her in a special study group. She credits this five-year health to three things: (1) daily exercise, which cleanses her lymphatic system through perspiration; (2) daily meditation; and (3) coming to terms with past-life challenges that have carried over into this lifetime.

You mean if I don't come to terms with my illness and work through this crap now I could have to deal with it in a future life? Or am I dealing with it now because of a past life? *"Breathe!"*

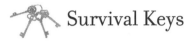 Survival Keys

* Move. Movement is life. Exercise ensures movement, which ensures life.

* Know your spirit is eternal. Your body changes from lifetime to lifetime like clothing.

* Trust you soul memory. Just as you have muscle memory, you have soul memory from past lifetimes. In order to progress, sometimes you must tie up your loose ends from previous lifetimes in this lifetime.

Chapter 38

9/11: LIGHTS, SMELLS, AND ACTION IN THE MIDDLE OF THE NIGHT

The only thing standing between you and your dreams is you.
Achieve by leading the way; don't stand in it.
— Kathleen O'Keefe-Kanavos

♥ *Affirmation:* Today I will look in the mirror and connect with my powerful self through the windows to my soul — my eyes.

Tuesday, September 11, 2001

Another year and a month has come and gone, and I had no reason to make an entry until now. Just when I feel I'm recovering more each day from the residual effects of surgery, chemotherapy, and radiation, it seems as though the world has begun to show symptoms of a severe illness. A different kind of cancer is spreading in a different type of body. As the universe's energy cries out warnings from other dimensions, some of us hear them but aren't sure what to do to help. What better way to gain attention than to shine a spotlight?

The spotlights over our bed turned on at 2:30 a.m. on September 8th, 2:45 a.m. on the 9th, and 3:00 a.m. on the 10th, followed by the smell of burnt flesh and coffee. The heat in our bedroom at those times was almost unbearable. If the heat continued to rise, combustion of some magnitude was a possibility. What was happening? The worst part was we had guests in the downstairs bedroom on the 8th, and we were afraid of what they would think of the smell and heat in the house. To our surprise, however, as soon as Peter and I stepped over the threshold of the bedroom, the smell and heat were gone. We discovered this each time we ran out of the bedroom looking for the source of both the heat and stench. Our immediate concern was that a short in the electrical system had activated the spotlight over our bed, which could result in a wall fire. The electrician could find nothing wrong. The problem was not in the wiring of our home. Was it in the wiring of the universe?

The morning of 9/11, I was awakened by a phone call from a tennis partner who is married to an Australian. We had planned to play tennis that morning.

"John just called me from work and yelled, 'Turn on the TV and see what's happening to your people,'" Nan shrieks over the phone, practically in tears. "So I did, and Kathy … we're being bombed! By jetliners!"

"Turn on the TV, Peter! Something's really wrong. We're being bombed," I say to my sleeping husband. He grunted something unintelligible, found the remote control hidden in the covers, and complied. We didn't need to flip to a specific news channel to see the carnage. Every channel was a news channel.

I couldn't believe my eyes. At first I thought it was all a terrible accident. Then I saw the deliberate action of the second plane. The blinding explosion as it hit the second tower of the World Trade Center. This was no mistake. But who would do such a horrible thing and why? Blazing buildings with burning people jumping to their deaths. The light, the heat, the smell, the horror of it all.

Two days later, I call Jeanne in Virginia Beach and tell her about the lights, heat, and smell we had experienced in our bedroom. Once I convince her that I'm quite recovered from my cancer treatments and eager to give something back to the universe for the spiritual support I received during my therapy, she invites me to astral travel with a large group of psychics. They've agreed on a specific time and day for their journey to where the Twin Towers had stood. Their goal is to help those who died but did not "cross over."

"Didn't cross over?" I ask. "How could they not cross over?"

"Because they don't know they're dead," Jeanne answers, "or they don't want to accept their fate." That thought gave me pause. I remembered Jack not crossing over because he still had some lessons to learn, but he did know he was dead, and he definitely wanted to cross over.

I've astral-traveled to hospitals to help friends in need, so why not help my fellow man or woman during this crucial time? If I can astral-travel to hospital rooms, I can go to the Towers; however, this is something I need to talk about with my guides, because I definitely don't want to go to site alone and without protection. How would I get back? How would I even know where to go? I've never been to the Towers in my life. If I decide to do this, and I haven't yet, it will be a big test and a turning point in my psychic/spiritual development. This questioning is the same uncertainty I experienced when I prepared to do my Dream Works with Kristin, the tiny coma patient. The answer I received then was *Believe*.

I wonder if the astral travel I did during my chemotherapy was a dry run for now. Maybe the chemo brain kept me too scrambled to rationalize that what I was attempting was supposedly impossible. Did all those paths lead to here and now, showing that we are all intertwined in the universe and connected by the Greater Power? Did my health challenges and chemotherapy bring these new intuitive abilities to the surface for a purpose? If I hadn't had cancer and chemo, would I still have had the same experiences preparing me for now? Would I have been in the frame of mind to develop those abilities, or would my biggest goal for the rest of my life still be to have fun in the sun playing tennis, scuba diving, and eating lunch with my friends? So many questions and so few answers, it's enough to make my head spin. The big question is: am I up to this? I have until September 15 to decide, only two days away.

It's Saturday, the day and time of the group astral-travel to the Twin Towers, and after meditating on the subject, I've decided to go. "They" got my attention. If they have shined a spotlight and turned up the heat in my world, it must be important for me to respond. After what the universe has given back to me, my life, how can I say no? I start my meditation by asking permission to go and help those in need. This is in keeping with the Rule of Permission. Help must be requested for permission to be given.

I recline on my bed and start my meditation by going to my special place, where I'm immediately met by a spirit guide in a belted and hooded cassock. It's the same guide who often took me to see Kristin and Tom. We're old friends now so I feel comfortable with him. Taking his hand, I tell him my fears about going and returning from this travel. "Please don't leave me there alone," are my last words as I find myself inside one of the towers and beside a woman who is seated on a step by a coffee cart. She's dressed in a full pleated skirt and dark blazer. She's young, mid-twenties, and has wavy dark hair that reaches her shoulders. "Who are you?" she asks, looking up from her coffee.

"Don't step over the light threshold," were the last words my guide said before disappearing. *What threshold?* I thought.

"Does anyone know we're down here?" the woman asks. I introduce myself and tell her I don't know. "I came down here to get some coffee and then I don't know what happened. Do you?" she asks, searching my face for a reaction, so I sit down beside her and tell her about the planes. I've always believed that if someone can ask a straight question, she can handle the answer; otherwise she wouldn't have been able to formulate the question in the first place.

"Am I dead?" she asks after a few moments.

"I think so," I reply. "Do you want me to call up the "light" so you can leave now?" I ask as gently as possible.

"I don't know if I want to go anywhere but home. I need to go home. Are you coming with me?" she asks, staring at the cup of to-go coffee in her hand.

"No. I'm not dead. I've come here with spirit-guides to help you." As if on cue, a bright light appears in the corner and she stands up and walks toward it. *"Don't step over the threshold,"* a voice beside me says, and I stop, turn, and see my guide in his cassock, pointing in the direction of the light and the woman. I had been walking without realizing it. Then the light, guide, and girl were gone.

Oh, that *threshold. Now I've got it! Where to next?* I think, gaining confidence from the realization that my guides are protecting me. I don't want to think about where I might be right now if my guide hadn't shown up before I reached that light. This is definitely not something anyone should attempt without guides.

An EXIT sign above a door catches my eye, and I walk through it ... into pandemonium. People descend the stairs on one side while firefighters, with all their heavy equipment, climb up the other. Despite their facemasks, the level of concentration in the eyes of some of the firefighters is unmistakable. *They don't know the towers have come down,* I think. They had one mission: to get to the floors above, where people were trapped and in need of rescue. Is this an energy rerun, or are these the actual spirits of the firefighters? How could I tell an energy rerun (the residual energy left from an experience acting like radio waves floating in space and picked up under the right circumstances) from an actual spirit who has not passed over?

"Move out of the way, ma'am," the winded voice of a firefighter says behind me. *He can see me!* That's confirmation. This is no rerun. Each time I appear in front of them and try to tell them they can't help anyone up here, that all the people are dead, they push past me with the same look of determination, annoyance, and concentration on their faces. I'd have been annoyed, too, had the tables been turned. Who was I to tell them their efforts were futile because everyone was already dead? I probably would have gone one step farther than they did and knocked me down the stairs, backwards.

Even though I didn't know how, I had pulled up the light downstairs. I hoped I could do it again. By now I realize that trying to talk these brave firefighters out of climbing those stairs is a waste of time, and I don't know long I can stay here in the time continuum, the plane between time and space and the living and the dead, a place consisting of the past, present, and future in a kind of quantum physics state of NOW. I also know that in their spirit state the firefighters can stay here indefinitely (something I didn't want for them), and knew I would soon have to return to my physical body. I still belonged to that time-dependent place called life. I keep expecting my guide to appear and say, *"Time to go"* and find myself back in my bedroom. *I need to call up that light,* I think, looking at the top of the stairs as the perfect place for it to appear ... and there it is!

"The people are inside that light up there," I said, reappearing for the third time in front of the leader while pointing to the top of the stairs. This light was the stairway or portal to the other side, either called up by the other group of psychics who astral-traveled here to help or by my spiritual guides. I wasn't sure who'd called it, but I was pretty sure I hadn't because as far as I knew, I didn't yet know how. But I planned to give it a try before I left. *Ask and ye shall receive* kept echoing in my mind.

The fireman looks at me, looks at the light, veers to the right, and leads the others into the bright portal beside the door to the 94th floor. *Oh, my God, did that just happen? That was way too easy. Am I allowed to say that?* I think, my hands over my mouth in disbelief. *Too late for that question now.* I continue up the stairs after the light folded in on itself, much like a tornado disconnecting from the earth and reentering the cloud from which it came. *Mustn't step over the threshold*, I repeat to myself, as much a reminder as a reassurance, and enter an office room where a woman anxiously sits alone at her desk.

"They will call me and tell me what to do. I'm waiting for instructions," she says as soon as she sees me, and points to the phone on her desk. Concentrating, I ask permission from my guides to open the room to the light portal. Within seconds, a large beam of light appears exactly as it had on the other floors. *I did it!* I turn my attention back to the woman at the desk and explain that the way out is through the light in the corner of the room, but she refuses to leave. She repeats that someone will call her with instructions, so she'll wait at her desk. "I wonder what's taking them so long to call," she says, and places her hand on the phone. After multiple attempts to persuade her to go into the light, I throw my hands up in despair and prepare to move on to someone else when Mom shows up. *Now I'm dreaming*, I think. *Someone wake me up!* I watch in disbelief as Mom walks over to the woman, smiles, takes her by the hand, and whispers in her ear. The woman stands up and walks to the light with Mom who, without so much as a single word to me, waves goodbye over her shoulder. Then the light, Mom, and the woman disappear, and I'm alone in the office room, not dreaming but definitely dumbfounded. *So, if this isn't a dream, I want to see where that plane crashed.*

From the stairway I enter a door numbered 103. The floor is filled with hanging metal illuminated by sparking live wires. Mohamed Atta is punching, kicking, and yelling at the jet instrument panel. He doesn't understand why he's still in the cockpit. He thinks he's still flying and that the jetliner isn't responding to his commands. Turning, he glares at me with crazed eyes, his face contorted with rage. *This man is mad, as mad as a rabid dog. And he can see me.* "Time to go!" my guide says, appearing beside me. In the next instant, I'm back in my bedroom with a pounding headache, drenched in perspiration.

An hour later the phone rings. It's Jeanne. "We felt you at the trade center." Her first concern was that I felt okay after so much spiritual work. She didn't want me to be overtired while still recovering from treatment. Our conversation lasted four hours as we compared notes and shared details that were astoundingly similar.

After finishing my story about Jeanne's invitation and the Twin Towers group travel, I tell Patricia over the phone: "So now, confident and empowered, I plan to go to the Pentagon and help the military personnel who haven't crossed over. Time is of the essence, and I hope I'll be fully rested by tomorrow. My heart is always with the military."

"Well, be sure to take your guides with you, dear. This is dangerous work you're doing," she warns. I promise I will. "And don't stay as long this time. I'm concerned about that headache you brought back last time." That might be a problem because I didn't look at my watch the last time; therefore I have no idea how long I was gone. After finding Atta, I was glad just to be home unharmed. What could be worse than he? I told God I would do anything He wanted as long as He protected me and sent me spiritual guides to take me and bring me back safely. He had done this, so I felt safe in my work now.

Again, I go to my special place, ask permission to help any Pentagon souls who might be in need, and ask my guides to accompany me. Seconds later, walking down a corridor I'm confronted by soldiers who ask what I'm doing in a high-security area. That's when I realize that I'm a non-uniformed civilian without a security badge and surrounded by uniformed soldier-spirits. In the military, some things never change. Realizing this astral trip is not going well, I ask my guides to take me out before I get hurt. Can an earthbound spirit harm me if I'm only astral-traveling to its location? I've learned that anything is possible in this realm, and I don't want to get that answer the hard way.

Once safely back in my special place, still shaken from the unexpected response of the soldiers, I ask my guides how I can safely help those soldiers, because it's obvious they don't realize they're dead. *"Dress in a uniform with your mind,"* they answer. Of course! Why didn't I think of that before going the first time? Now dressed as a colonel, I return to the Pentagon and simply order them into the light. Even from the other side they follow a commanding officer's orders, so what had begun as my most difficult challenge ended up being the easiest. When I called Patricia and told her, she laughed. "Your guides are clever."

They appear to know us well and can certainly shed light on dark situations.

 ## Survival Keys

* Get an astral travel guide. Astral travel is the kind of spiritual work that's not for everyone and should be done under the supervision of a trusted instructor with spiritual guides.

* Take the time to get to know your guides. It takes years to develop a relationship with spirit guides, but it's so rewarding.

* Learn astral travel. Dreams are a great natural place to start.

Chapter 39

WARS AND BATTLES, ABOVE AND BELOW

There is only one way to happiness, and that is to cease worrying about things which are beyond the power of our will.
— Epictetus (AD 55–AD 135)

♥ *Affirmation:* I give out love, and it is returned to me multiplied.

I still dream lucid dreams, but they seem to have less to do with healing me and more to do with healing the world. Perhaps we are ill because we're a reflection of the world, or is the world ill because it's a reflection of us? One cannot heal without the other because the interdependence of life binds us together, much like the body and spirit.

Last night I dreamed of Florida. I named this dream "A Phone Call from John and Winston." In it I tell people in a waiting room that I had placed a call to my father and was waiting for an answer. On the far wall of this room, the dream shifts to a movie of armies of young men training in a wet, boggy area with warm waters and canals. An old Green Beret boyfriend of mine is training them to roll a big boulder up a steep hill. I turn my attention away from the wall when a boy appears outside the door and says, "I don't know if I can be in a room with people who are forty." I tell him it's okay. He smiles, enters the room, and waits with everyone.

An answering machine turns on and a man's voice says, "This is John and Winston returning your call."

"That sounded like a used-car dealership," I say to the people. My attention is again pulled to the far wall where I see a birds-eye view of a desert with rocky, treeless mountains like the Arizona desert. A large mushroom cloud rises from the ground, followed by the explosive sound of a bomb.

At that moment the three overhead spotlights awaken both Peter and me in our bedroom by turning on so brightly they hum from the electrical overload. (The same spotlights that kept turning on before 9/11.) The intense heat and the odor of burning flesh and coffee grounds are again so overpowering that Peter jumps out of bed and declares, "That's it! I've had it! I'm sleeping in the other bedroom."

As he steps over our bedroom threshold he stops and begins to hop in and out of the bedroom. He looked like he was doing an Irish jig. This alarmed me until he declared, "The heat and smell are only in our bedroom. It's cool in the hallway. Are you coming?" he asks and sprints down the hallway. The time on the clock is 3:43 a.m. *God*, I think as I follow Peter into the other room, *I pray we don't have a bomb dropped on us*. I don't want a bomb dropped on *anyone*, but I really don't want one dropped on me. I don't think that's a selfish thought, just strong survival instinct, and right now, with what I'm going through medically, my survival instinct is at its highest level ever.

On the evening news, at 4:43 p.m., President Bush announces opening attacks on Afghanistan and says about forty nations are involved in the antiterrorism coalition including our greatest ally, Great Britain … Sir Winston Churchill and John F. Kennedy? There seem to be an awful lot of fours going on here. Four is the spiritual number for the earth.

Interpretation: This is a precognitive dream about kismet and impending war. But whose fate is it? War, even a just war, is viewed (as a movie on the far wall) as an oxymoron, perhaps necessary in defense but futile in the long run. It's a no-win situation because wars are won when battles and lives are lost at the hands of commanders, as seen with the soldiers bogged down in swamps or being treated like the Greek mythological figure Sisyphus, pushing his boulder up a steep hill only to have it roll back down. (My war with cancer was won when the lives of my cells were sacrificed for the greater good of my body, which is still trying to recover.) Soldiers bogged down in water and bogs while being trained to do futile tasks is a duality of spirit and earth. What we do on earth affects all the realms, because earth and heaven are intertwined. The saying "as it is above so shall it be below" works both ways. Are John and Winston aware of what's going on here and answering us across time and space? Do they represent only England and the United States, or more? Even better, are John and Winston going to help? It would make sense that they would have permission to help if we truly were all part of the Greater Power. Is the Greater Power taking sides? If so, whose side is She on, because I believe I saw the future when that bomb went off. I'm left with more questions than answers, leading me to believe it was a message in a dream state given in the room between realms that I've visited many times. It was a warning of impending war.

After rereading my dream and recalling the unrest in our home, it occurs to me that I'm extremely lucky to be married to Peter. Any other man would have run out of the house and down the drive-way — barefoot and half naked — in the early morning hours, never to be heard from again except through a divorce attorney. Yes, we truly are a match made in heaven. I wonder if Peter still wants to soak in a bathtub full of stuff to be able to better commune with the other side, or if he thinks he has heard enough now. I think I would soak in that bathtub not to be quite as connected with the other side, but this seems to be out of our hands. I don't understand how this information from the other side can be helpful to the world. What can I do? I'm just one relatively insignificant person, not an army. And who is going to listen to me? I could be crazy.

I present Jeanne with these same questions and she has an interesting response: "By bringing the future into the present accompanied with physicality, such as heat, smell, and lights, the opportunity presents itself to change that future." Most likely many other sensitives had similar experiences, and passing the word enables a change for the better, because it couldn't get much worse. The more this dream is talked about the more likely it is to effect change. In other words, change the future by talking about it now.

It's been one month and two days since 9/11. Jeanne's explanation of the purpose of the dreams of war has encouraged me to call together all the psychics, spiritualists, sensitives, and healers I can find on Cape Cod. I now know the importance of telling as many people as possible about the war dreams so as to spread the word. I was acquainted with a couple of spiritualists (people who commune with the dead) and simply put out *the word*. And the word traveled throughout the spiritual community, culminating in our first Gathering.

Our first monthly meeting consisted of eleven people: a spiritual · ist who volunteers at the local hospital and helps dying patients "pass over" without fear or being alone; six Reiki masters who explained how they were treating more people than ever for stress and sleep disorders; two healers who use chakra color therapy; a healer who uses footbaths to cleanse the body, and me.

Nancy, one of the spiritualists who worked in New York during the week, told of feelings she had of spirits trying to insinuate themselves into her body like a succubus. She felt they were desperate to get home to their families, refusing to accept the fact that they were dead. Others in the group then said they were having similar experiences. We called this the *succubus syndrome* and used our collective energy fields to increase individual protective energy fields and teach members of the group how to close their chakras when necessary. Nancy said, "If I had gone to a regular psychiatrist with these feelings and stories, I would either have been medicated or committed. We need other people who are experiencing similar phenomena to share with." Many in the room nodded their agreement.

Thus began our first of many Gatherings. We started with a discussion time or psychic group therapy, sharing any recent unusual experiences, and then broke into small groups and took turns using different healing practices on each other. It felt great when they put their healing hands on me. I always sleep better the night after a Gathering.

Most of my dreams still deal with world events. This takes my mind off myself but at the same time it worries me to have to worry about the world. I just finished a physical war, and now I have to witness another war outside my body that's just as deadly. A worldwide anger is spreading out of control and destroying everything in its path.

I know how important it is to make our own reality, and I'm trying to keep a peaceful inner being, but it's difficult when I'm bombarded by destruction. I still try not to watch the news at night before I go to bed, but sometimes news comes to me in my sleep.

Dream: R-I-A-D and *Catcher in the Rye*

At 3:53 a.m. this morning, I awoke to the aroma of baking onion bread and the sound of a child's laughter. At 4:00 a.m. I fell back to sleep and dreamed of attending a university in Munich, Germany, where I actually attended high school. In one of the classes I ask the professor, "Who is behind this latest terrorism?" He answers, "Riyadh" and leaves. As I walk back to the bus, I see some spirit guides. I've been repeating Catcher in the Rye *to myself in order to remember* Riyadh *when I awaken. Walking over to the guides, I tell them I need to know who's responsible for this latest terrorism. They say the word "Riyadh" and slowly spell it aloud for me. "I can't remember all those letters," I say impatiently. "They don't make any sense. Spell it so I can remember it, like CIA or FBI, or I won't remember it to take back." A guide takes me to a sandy spot in a dessert, puts a pointed stick in my hand, and holding my hand, writes in the sand, in large letters, R-I-A-D.*

Interpretation: This is a precognitive guided dream. The university is a duality, both ethereal and earthly. I went to high school in Munich, Germany, where I read *Catcher in the Rye* by J. D. Salinger. In my dream I used *Catcher in the Rye* as a means to bring back the dream information, yet the similarities between the book and the terrorists was astounding. I asked a direct question and my instructor and guides gave me a direct answer in three different ways to help me remember the information. The source of the terrorism was Riyadh, Saudi Arabia.

Other than my frightening dreams of the present and future, life is a party again. I had a combination birthday-tennis-team-Christmas party-2001 and invited all my newfound friends on Cape Cod. At

2:00 a.m., as Peter and I walked through the house to lock up and turn off Christmas lights, we found two people fast asleep in the library. Life is good again!

Survival Keys

* Manifest from dreams. It's important to make your own reality by manifesting the positive life of your dreams.

* Change the ending of your lucid dreams and change your future for the better, forever. The same holds true for dreams about the world.

Chapter 40

BECKY'S SECOND WAR

I would rather walk with God in the dark
than go alone in the light.
— Mary Gardiner Brainard (1837–1905)

♥ *Affirmation:* I will see and understand the big picture.

Becky has given me grave news: her cancer has returned. "So they took my blood and made a chemotherapy infusion out of it that should have worked, but it didn't. It just made me really sick. Now I'm on my third chemo and it's worse than the others. Plus, Dr. Harold is doing radiation on me at the same time I'm taking the chemo. He's hoping to shrink the tumor in my neck with this double-whammy treatment. I'm so tired of being sick and tired and in pain."

I listen to Becky describe her latest torture and struggle not to cry into the phone. This was the chemo treatment Dad had spoken of the night I told him I had cancer. I guess he knew what he was talking about because they're using it on Becky. This is horrible! A nightmare on steroids, but I can't express my emotions; I have to stay positive for Becky. In order to not let her hear the fear and grief in my voice as I reassure her with Dad's insight, I ball my fingers up into a fist, squeeze my nails into my palm, and have an "Aha moment" — this is why people physically harm themselves when their emotional pain is so great. The physical pain grounds you and helps you deal with grief.

It all started when I called Becky to wish her a Merry Christmas, hoping to laugh and joke like we always did. Instead, she told me her cancer was back with a vengeance. (*Merry fucking Christmas!*) I've been so upset it's taken me a week to write about it. Her words hit me like a ton of bricks. I had to sit down, steady my voice, and struggle not to sob while I spoke with her. No one should ever have to say the words "my cancer is back." Once in a lifetime is more than enough, twice is criminal, torturous, and cruel. I don't even know if I could get the words out of my mouth if I were in Becky's shoes. It should be universally illegal. I remember holding Mom in my arms after she found out her cancer was back. I wish I could have reached through that telephone line and held Becky. I wish she could have reached through and held me because I'm just as frightened for myself as for her. If this can happen to Mom and Becky, it can happen to anyone. *Shhh… don't think such things!* my inner parents and grandparents chide. *The children are already upset…"I can't help it!"* I answer. *"Will this nightmare ever end!?"*

Becky had had a scare about six months ago. A full body scan showed a spot on her liver.

"The doctors did some other tests, then told me the spot was nothing. "You're fine, Becky," they said. Well, I guess I wasn't. Everyone in our radiation group is doing great except me," she sobbed.

"This disease is going to kill me," Mom had said when her cancer returned, and it did. Now I could hear that same terror in Becky's voice. Is it a premonition?

"Listen, Becky, we went through this before and we can do it again. It is what it is, so let's put on our boxing gloves and get to it. You're not alone. I'm here for you and with you," I said bravely quaking in my winter boots from fear, not cold.

Being as close as sisters, we had finally discussed my intuitive abilities in one of our monthly talks, and Becky was okay with it. One day she brought up the subject and it just sort of evolved from there. The fact that I saw ghosts didn't make her love me less.

"Do you really see people who have died when you're on the other side?" Becky asked.

"Yes, I do. They're really there. I've seen them and had confirmation about them from other family members who didn't know me or know what I do," I replied, afraid to imagine why she was asking this question now. "This life is not the end. It's only a transition between all our other lives, and we all have family and friends waiting for us on the other side of death's thin veil. Our bodies all have to die sooner or later, Becky. That's the rule here on earth, but our souls live on. And from what I've seen of life on the other side while visiting the sick in hospitals and speaking with spirits visiting them, they throw fabulous welcome-home parties when we die. I mean SERIOUS PARTIES."

It broke my heart to have this conversation, so I cried on the inside as I cheerfully laughed on the outside. This was a dose of reality for both of us. I knew these answers could give Becky a different kind of hope if things took a turn for the worse. Maybe trying to help someone pretend she's going to live forever is not as comforting as explaining that in the natural course of life and death, she is never alone. There's more comfort in peace of mind than unrealistic expectations of living forever. It is not a failure to let go and let God take over. Like Mom said, "None of us are getting off this planet alive."

"Well, I'd rather die later than sooner, because I still have things to do in this life. I'm not ready to give up this fight," Becky stated emphatically.

"I don't want you to go yet either, so I'll fight with you. I'm calling a prayer group that does Reiki. I believe they helped me. You hang in there, Becky; they're coming out with new treatments every six months. I'll call you from California in a couple of weeks, okay?"

"Kathy, I don't think I have six months left. I don't know if I have six weeks. Call me."

I've had a wonderful time traveling to California and Europe to visit old tennis friends and family, but thoughts of Becky and her renewed cancer battle crept into my mind day and night. I wish I could write good things about what I feel she's going through, but I can't. I know the path of life we walk is our own, but we shared such an important part of that path. Other than doing Reiki on her every night and praying for her, I don't know what else to do, so this is where I take a leap of faith and let go and let God. Becky's been asleep when I've called. Sometimes, I wake up in the middle of the night and, after calculating the time difference between Europe, California, and New

England, know that she's thinking about me. We were still connected at the heart despite time and distance. I left messages with John so she'd know I was thinking of her, that she's constantly on my mind.

The Reiki group said Becky's colors and energy are not good. They see the same thing I see: Becky's aura is fading. It's not green and yellow anymore, it's a pale gray. I'm so worried about her. Even if it means waking her, I'm calling Becky tomorrow when I get home. I need to speak with her.

"Hi, John, it's Kathy. How is Becky doing with her new chemo? Can she talk?"

"Kathy, I tried to call you, but your cat sitter said you were out of the country," John says, voice filled with grief. "Becky died last week. She asked for you."

Survival Keys

* Know you are in transition. This life is only a transition between all our other lives.

* Embrace death. In order to live life to the fullest we must embrace death as a friend.

* Look forward to reunion. We all have family and friends waiting for us on the other side of death's thin veil.

* Know that you are never alone.

Chapter 41

COMING TO GRIPS AND EXHALING

We could never learn to be brave and patient
if there were only joy in the world.
— Helen Keller (1880–1968)

♥ *Affirmation:* I now let go and let God.

It's been six months since my last entry. This sounds like a confession and maybe it is, because I feel guilty. Emotions don't always make sense. It's taken me this long to come to terms with Becky's death and write about my feelings. Avoidance is not a recommended form of therapy, but sometimes we have to do what we have to do to survive mentally and emotionally. I've heard it said that time heals all. I guess I needed time. Over time the numbness of shock is replaced by pain. But which is less painful... a broken bone or a broken heart?

Why did Becky die while I lived? I have survivor's guilt that I've heard officers talk about. Why did they survive the war that killed their friends? Surviving a health crisis has taught me about the element of life as applied to the "Periodic Table of Humans": Norms become less predictable as life becomes more desirable because of the presence of spirit. I'll bet that's not in any science book. Spirit is seldom studied by science because it's in constant flux. What is its anatomy? If you want to see it just look in the mirror. The eyes are the windows to the soul.

I had an MRI last month and it showed I was healthy, just like the one a year ago. I feel really guilty writing about all my good fortune, so I'll stop for now.

"I think we can cut back to seeing you to once a year, Kathy," Dr. Barkley says from his little black stool during my six-month Tuesday checkup. "We discussed you at our last meeting, and we're all in agreement with this, if you are."

"All" referred to my three doctors who had slowly increased my time between checkups from once a week to once a month. That stretched to twice a year, and now I've graduated to ONCE A YEAR!

"That's great!" I answer. Once a year versus every six months equals more freedom and fewer blood tests. I had just jumped over a big hurdle. The biggest hurdle will be staying cancer-free for five years, but today feels like a big turning point.

"Okay, you can get dressed."

"Uh, what about my blood test?" I ask, like a naughty child waiting for the scolding she knows she deserves and can't believe was forgotten.

"You don't need one, you're healthy. See you in a year."

I sprint down the hall and pull on my clothing as I run, in case he changes his mind.

It's mid-August, and the summer has been gorgeous. I've played tennis, lunched, and lived the good life with family and friends again. My calendar is filled with joyful social events including the monthly Gatherings. Right now life is wonderful and I pray it will last. That old saying, "you don't know what you've got until it's gone" has been indelibly etched in my mind by my past. Perhaps in the future, if I ever become complacent about my health, I'll remind myself of what I once more have but could have lost my life.

There are times in one's life that are so profound that they take on a persona of their own, such as "before and after," much like before and after WWII and 9/11. Mine is "Before Cancer" and "After Cancer" — BC and AC. What a kick in the pants!

Crisis affects the whole family. As hard as I tried, it was difficult to separate my treatment life from my private one because the demands of those therapies and ensuing follow-ups have determined the shape of my emotional sphere, melding both lives together to become a tumultuous time for everyone within that sphere. My emotional ups and downs coincided with my medical appointments and tests. I'm still anxious about every ache and pain in my body, fearing the worst. I try hard to control my mind and look forward to the day my fears subside and a headache is just a headache and a sore muscle is normal again.

Winston Churchill wrote, "When the notes of life ring false, men should correct them by referring to the tuning fork of death. It is when that clear menacing tone is heard that the love of life grows keenest in the human heart."

His words ring true on multiple levels, both literally and figuratively, because my nightly meditations end with angels going over my body with a tuning fork to keep in check my other "tuning fork" of life and death: cancer. The life I took for granted or complained about before my cancer tuning fork struck its "clear and menacing tone" has now become very precious to me. When you think life is as bad as it can get, think about how much worse the alternative, death, could be, and get a grip. I guess I've been duly, painfully, adjusted and tuned.

It's amazing how many women I run into who've gone through a health crisis and survived to talk about it, which is so educational. One such case is a new tennis friend from the Friday night round-robin mixed doubles. Irene heard that I had just completed treatment and wanted to congratulate me. She is nine months ahead of me on the road of recovery and doing great. One thing led to another and, as so often happens, we ended up comparing notes.

"I saw this program on TV," Irene says, "and it caught my attention because it was about breast cancer and how one of the most often missed symptoms is severe itching inside the breast. Well, I had a healthy mammogram eight months before my itching began, but after seeing that program I asked for a second mammogram. A five-centimeter tumor was found on the underside of my breast."

"Did the first mammogram miss the tumor?" I was captivated by the story.

"No. The tumor wasn't there. It was a lobular tumor and covered most of the underside of my breast. It was too large for a lumpectomy, so I had a mastectomy and reconstructive surgery done at the same time. When they checked my lymph nodes, three were affected, so most of them were removed. Now when I play tennis I wear a compression sleeve to keep my arm from swelling from lymphedema. I used a doctor in Maryland who specialized in TRAM-flap surgery using the 'skin-saving method.' All the breast tissue was scraped from the skin that was saved for reconstructive surgery, and my nipple was rebuilt in one operation. After everything healed, I went back and had areolas tattooed to complete my new breast. You can't even see my breast scar because it's under the breast fold — and I got a great tummy tuck at the same time."

We had had the same chemotherapy, but Irene went on to have Taxotere, very similar to Taxol, the drug the CSRA tests said wouldn't work for me. Ilene said it really made her sick. "The nurses told me to just sleep as much as possible, that sleep was a means of recovering, so I did. I slept all the time."

"Did you get neuropathy from the Taxotere?" I wanted to know how Irene held onto the tennis racquet if she still suffered from it.

"Yes, but it faded within months. What hasn't gone away is the constant tearing in my left eye. The doctor says it's a very rare side effect of the chemotherapies."

It's a small price to pay for life, but that's easy for me to say — I don't have a weepy eye. It puts my trauma and fears in perspective.

One thing we did have in common was "barometric pressure pain." Whenever there's a climate change, we know about it before the Weather Channel. All the irradiated bones and surgery sites in our bodies telegraph the storm's distance and ETA (estimated time of arrival).

After Peter and I play mixed doubles tennis today with another couple, we decide to go to a wonderful little bakery in the basement of an old building in Dennis for scones and cream. The aromas that greet us through the screen door are absolutely delicious and elicit a mouthwatering response similar to Pavlov's drooling dogs. While Peter and Jim pay for the scones and coffee, Jan and I sit at the little round 1960s aluminum table and weave-pattern chairs. We spread napkins on the chairs so we won't suffer from waffle thighs. Just as I settle comfortably on my napkins, Jan asks me if I know of any psychics who could give her a reading on her ailing mother who's been falling often. "I'm afraid mother won't last more than two weeks," she says with tears in her eyes. I was surprised about Jan's mother and surprised that Jan would ask me if I knew any psychics. I had never mentioned my spiritual work to her or any of my other tennis friends. It's very anxiety inducing to give readings to friends rather than to strangers, because I'll see my friends again, most likely at tennis, whereas I might never see a stranger again. I've always had a fear of friends thinking that I'd converse with their long-dead relatives during a tennis match, resulting in a Vaudevillian scene: "Your serve is out," my friend says. "No, it's not," I reply — "and your great-great-grandmother agrees with me!"

Putting my fears aside, I give Jan a reading right then, in a crowded pastry shop. A thin spirit with short shiny blond hair appears beside Jan, but only I can see her. She identifies herself as Anna. (When Jan later described Anna to her conservative Bostonian mother, her mom immediately confirmed Anna as a deceased childhood friend.) During the reading, Anna laughs and says, "Jan's mother is going to be fine and live many more years, but I'm far more worried about Jan running herself ragged caring for her demanding mom."

As Anna slowly disappears, two of the mother's spirit guides appear and give a second reading with specific medical information. They say Jan's mother has been overmedicated, causing a number of problems including dehydration, which affects her balance. They also say that the cause of the mother's leg pain is a hairline fracture in her left hip from falling, and that she should get a new doctor. The guide sys, "Butler," then disappears, ending the reading in the busy shop.

The following day a Dr. Butler phones Jan and asks if he can take over her mother's case. New test results have shown that the mother is dehydrated from overmedication and has a hairline fracture in her left hip that was missed in previous X-rays but found in an MRI. Jan's mother began physical therapy to walk again. The reading not only helped the mother, who was thrilled to hear from Anna, but also gave reassurance that best friends on the other side do look out for us during times of need and can give us helpful information.

A few nights later, during a dream, the phone line sends an unusual and lifesaving message. My spirit guides dress up as doctors dressed as circus clowns. Well, my life is a three-ring circus.

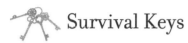 ## Survival Keys

* ✳ Know you are a spiritual being from another dimension inhabiting a human body on earth.

* ✳ Trust in an answer. Your dreams are your ET (eternal teacher) phoning home. Someone will answer.

* ✳ Forgive yourself. Survivor's guilt is normal and, like grief, is a form of love.

* ✳ Take care of your spirit and it will take care of you. The Periodic Table of Humans states: Norms become less predictable as life becomes more desirable because of the presence of spirit.

Chapter 42
VOICES VS. DOCTORS, AGAIN

Yesterday is gone. Tomorrow has not yet come.
We have only today. Let us begin.
— Mother Teresa (1910–1997)

♥ *Affirmation:* I treasure every day I am living.

I'm filled with anxiety as I wait to be called to have my mammogram read in front of me. This moment reminds me of the dream I had years ago about being on *the list* and waiting to be called by *the doctors*. Was my life imitating a dream again, or was it the other way around?

This is one reason I transferred my mammograms from the Faulkner Hospital to the Dana-Farber where a trained physician goes over the results with me the same day. The second reason is the hospital computers are linked, so the results are immediately sent to all my doctors.

I don't recall being this nervous during previous mammograms; in fact, I remember feeling quite confident. Now I'm having difficulty breathing and feel cold and clammy — symptoms of a classic anxiety attack. It doesn't help that I can't change out of the hospital gown until the technicians are certain they have all the mammography shots they need. They've already called me back in once to take more. Is something wrong?

Perhaps I already know the answer, because I think I've been hearing unintelligible voices whispering in the background of my mind all day. Fortunately, I haven't seen any guides. I need to focus on positive things like last week's healthy gynecological exam, negative Pap smear, and ultrasound performed on my uterus and ovaries. My bone-density and blood tests were all great too, so why the hell am I so frightened? Maybe I'm experiencing free-floating anxiety stemming from all the 9/11 anniversary concerns, or maybe it's déjà vu all over again, only it's still in this lifetime. What do you call that? A voice distracts me from my mental babble. "The doctor is ready to see you, Ms. Kanavos."

"Congratulations, Ms. Kanavos!" the doctor says, turning to greet me while seated on a stool with wheels, not unlike Dr. Barkley's. *Must be a doctor thing.* My eyes strain to adjust to the dark cubbyhole of an office. The walls display multiple backlit mammography photos of breasts; my name is printed in bold capital letters on the lower corners. No doubt about it, they were mine. "You have a healthy mammogram. I'll send the results downstairs to your doctor. You may get dressed now."

With a sigh of relief, I look closely at the mammogram. My relief was short-lived when a voice countered, *"Don't believe it! Look right here and here." Oh, shit, where did you come from? Here we go again! Tell me you're not here!* I thought, pulling my gown closer around my trembling body as I stared at the hooded guide standing beside me. My breasts are under attack again. The light at the end of the tunnel really is a train that just blew its whistle.

"Are you sure?" I ask the doctor. "What about over here?" I say, pointing to an area on the mammogram as if an unseen hand were guiding my finger.

Again the doctor faces me, looks surprised, pauses, then turns back and points to the mammogram displaying the scar tissue from the lumpectomy on the right breast, then to the left breast and replies with a reassuring smile, "See, everything is healthy. You are healthy." And as if to send the message home (or dismiss me), he turns again and shakes my hand. "You can get dressed, now." I look beside me. The guide is gone.

"Yeah, okay. Thanks. Bye." *I guess the voices were my imagination,* I argue with myself. *But what about the guide who orbed into the room? More imagination?*

As soon as I walk up to Peter in the waiting room he asks me what's wrong. "Nothing's wrong, Bunny. The doctor read the mammogram and said it was another healthy one." The look of confusion on his face is the result of the positive verbal language he was hearing juxtaposed with my negative vibrations. After this great news, I should have been doing cartwheels up and down the room, *happiness* written all over my face. But it wasn't. I didn't want to alarm Peter with my guide's visit when things seemed to be going so well. "But I think I need an MRI. I'm going downstairs to talk to Dr. Harold and ask him to make an appointment for me."

Dr. Harold was waiting for me when I walked into the waiting room. "Dr. Goopka called and said you were on your way down here, Kathy." *That's odd. How did Dr. Goopka know?* We both agree that you're suffering from anxiety. Go home. You're healthy."

Later that evening, while lying in my bathtub, I poured water over my head while I pored over the day's events. I feel cheated. I should be overjoyed to see a healthy mammogram, yet, once again, which do I believe, my voices or my eyes? It's not like last time when I examined my mammogram in Dr. Kritchen's office. No one could read that one because it looked like a waxing crescent moon. This time the image was so clear even I could read it, so why shouldn't I believe it? And if I believe my voices over proof, how do I convince my doctors again? How do I convince myself again?

Peering up through the skylight, I search the night and see the full moon peering down at me. It's been so long since I even noticed the moon, but there he was, my friend, the man in the moon. "Where have you been? Look, Mom, it's our moon. I've had so much to think about today. I'm so afraid that history is repeating itself and I don't know what to do. I feel like my life is spiraling out of control and I'm the butt of some deadly joke — like a sign has been taped to my back reading, PLEASE KICK ME! I'M DOWN AND DON'T KNOW IT YET! I want so badly to believe the doctors and tell my voices to leave me alone. I've had enough voices and bad news in one lifetime. But I don't think I can. I don't think I should. I don't think I dare."

So while soaking in my candlelit bathroom, I tell Mom everything I was hearing and feeling beneath the light of the silvery moon. After my long one-sided conversation, I decide to sleep on all the information before deciding whether to believe the medical results or my guide. Sleep. That's what I really need, because when I awaken the real nightmare always resumes.

Dream: "Scary Clown"

Two guides in hooded cassocks pull me from my dream through a pop-up and into a brightly lit white hospital room where a third guide holds up mammograms in one hand and points to them with the other. She wears a white medical coat over her robe and matching white hat and clogs rather than the customary hood and brown sandals. Reluctantly, I step closer, stare at the mammogram, and see nothing but my name printed in black block letters on the bottom. She holds one plate closer, points to it again, and grimaces like a scary circus clown. Then she instantly turns into one, wearing a clown suit with huge red shoes and nose and a curly orange hair. "Wake up! This is a nightmare!"

I don't need a dream dictionary to decipher last night's precognitive guided nightmare. I got it! It made me decide to believe my voices over my eyes. Now, how do I win over the doctors? I'll find out tomorrow with Dr. Harold. Again, I'll be armed with feathers in my puny war chest while he'll have a chest full of undisputable medical evidence. Same feather, same life-threatening condition, different doctors. How weird is this? Someone wake me the fuck up!

"Kathy, all of your mammograms are healthy, as are your blood tests and physical exams," Dr. Harold says when I turn up for my appointment. *This really is déjà vu!* Have I suddenly been transported back in time to four and a half years ago in Dr. Wagner's office? I think I need to pinch myself, or better yet pinch Dr. Harold whose voice has risen an octave in exasperation.

"Your bone densities and gynecological exams have been great, too. You name it, Kathy, you've had the tests done and you are healthy! You don't need an MRI. It's not hospital policy to give MRIs without a good reason. They can give you false positives."

"I don't trust mammograms, and with good reason. I've had negative mammograms that should have been positive. I'd rather follow up on a false positive than die from a missed one, so I want an MRI, too," the attorney holding the feather in me counters.

He studies me with his blue eyes. "Okay, tell my secretary to make the MRI appointment for you, and I'll see you in a year," Dr. Harold says and closes my chart and the door behind him.

Well that wasn't nearly as bad as I thought it would be, I think as I hop down from the examining table. *I hope the rest is this easy.*

"I'm sorry, nothing is available at this time. I'll keep trying and call you," the secretary says.

"How soon do you think something will open up? I don't want to wait too long."

"I don't know. When it does I'll call you."

A month later I was back in the doctor's office. When I called to inquire about my MRI appointment, the secretary told me that she couldn't get me one this year, and that since more than thirty days had passed since my previous request, I needed another appointment for a new request. "Why must I get another appointment for an MRI prescription from the doctor for the same prescription I haven't been able to fill because appointments have been unavailable? I don't need another MRI prescription, just an appointment."

"That is the policy."

So here I am again. I don't know how I'll get this MRI, but I will get it or sleep here on the floor — and I'm not kidding.

"MRIs can give false positives, and your mammogram in August was fine," Dr. Harold says again, as I get dressed. I'm really getting tired of this crap. What the hell am I doing here wasting precious time? I can tell he's tired of it, too. He's not smiling. *Touché!*

"It also says the MRI you had scheduled last year was canceled because of a problem?"

"Yes. But it was never rescheduled, because there were no openings or cancellations. That's why getting one now is so important to me. The day of my MRI appointment last year, I told the MRI people I needed an emergency IV nurse for my difficult veins. They told me it was hospital policy to try to insert the dye needle first. If they were unsuccessful then they would call for backup. Well, after four unsuccessful attempts they called for backup, but none was available because of an emergency in the emergency room. My time was cutting into the next MRI patient's, so I had to leave for my other appointments with Dr. Kritchen, Dr. Barkley, and you. I asked your secretary then to please call for a new MRI date but she couldn't get me one. The MRI center said to keep calling in case there was a cancellation. Now the same thing is happening. It's been two years since I've had an MRI."

"So why do you want one now?"

Didn't I just explain that? An explanation of "the voices in my head told me so" along with "I had this scary guided clown dream" would not get me my MRI, but they might get me committed for life, which, if I don't get that MRI soon, might not be very long. Life's a bag of shit and giggles. Right now, I want to let out a crazy giggle and hit someone over the head with the remaining contents.

"Okay. Go out and have my secretary make the appointment for you."

YES!

"We don't make those appointments," the secretary says from behind her desk. "We didn't make the last one."

"Well, who did, and why are you telling me this now? Haven't you been calling for my appointment?" I ask. "I know you said the schedule was full so you weren't able to get me an appointment last year, but I really need this MRI, now."

"Well, try Dr. Barkley's office on the ninth floor and see if they can make the appointment for you," the secretary says, turning away to answer the phone. Peter and I look at each other and head for the elevator.

Nine minutes and nine floors later, I get the same answer from Dr. Barkley's secretary: "We never requested your other MRIs. That was done somewhere else in a different office. Try Dr. Harold again, because I believe he requested the last one, or maybe Dr. Kritchen's office on the third floor requested it."

Twelve minutes and nine floors later I'm back two floors below ground level in nuclear medicine and not in a good mood!

"I think this is called a runaround, and I'm not going to any more floors or doctor's offices," I hiss at Dr. Harold's secretary who is safely behind her desk. I lean forward, making direct eye contact, and smile at her to make my point. "I want you to make that appointment for me, and I'm not — repeat, NOT — leaving this office till I have it!" As she opens her mouth to protest, I hold up my hand. "You have my records in front of you. If you didn't make the last one, see who did, and call them. NOW!"

Apparently one of the other secretaries went looking for Dr. Harold, because the door to the waiting room opens and there he is, not looking at all happy. As far as I'm concerned that makes two of us.

"I don't want any more runaround," I announce to him and anyone else within earshot. "I want that appointment, and I don't care if it can give me a false positive." I hold my angel feather tightly in my hand. I know it's invisible to them, but it's very real to me.

"Okay, Kathy, but it's not hospital policy to do an MRI without a good reason."

"Which is more important," I ask. "Policy or patients? You want a good reason? Okay! I had multiple mammograms that missed my previous stage-two tumor that had spread to a lymph node. If it had it been caught earlier with a MRI it might not have invaded my lymph node. Cancer didn't show up in my blood tests and couldn't be felt. What better reason do you need? I am not leaving this office without an MRI. I will lie down here on your floor, kick my feet, and scream like a child who's had her candy taken away. You'll have to call security to drag me out by my feet, and I'll be dialing Channel 2 news as I'm dragged."

The feather wins again! The appointment is scheduled for December 14, two months and five days before my birthday. (More unwelcome déjà-damn-vu.) Three months have passed since my voices returned. Well, I have an appointment now, so I guess I shouldn't complain. Yes, I should! The U.S. doesn't have socialized medicine and is not a third-world country with third-world health practices. No one should have to fight this hard to live. Isn't that what doctors are for? Shouldn't they fight for me, or at least be fighting with me? Why do I feel like I'm always running the race of life alone as the medical staff stands on the sidelines laughing at me as I sprint by? Am I just feeling sorry for myself or do I have a legitimate gripe?

I leave for California on January 16 for a month. I need to really enjoy my upcoming vacation after that MRI because my voices only stopped their demands and took off those clown suits when I got my appointment. For now, silence is golden.

Two days before the MRI, I receive an early morning phone call. "Is this Kathleen Kanavos? This is the MRI center calling. One of our technicians had a bad accident and is in the hospital. Would you mind terribly if we rescheduled you for Tuesday, January fourteenth? Sorry."

What was I going to say? "No! Make her drag her broken butt in for my MRI!"

"Sure. Don't you have anything sooner? I've been waiting quite a while for this test."

"We don't. Thank you so much for understanding. Goodbye." CLICK.

If it's delayed again, I'll go to the hospital and perform that MRI on myself.

I've decided to put this out of my mind and have a nice Christmas and New Year's, just like five years ago, in case things are again not good. (History just keeps repeating itself.) That's the silver lining. When you don't learn from history you are doomed to repeat it. I've learned that my guides wouldn't be helping help me if I were meant to die. If the results are what I think they will be, this is beyond déjà vu, history, and synchronicity — it's Divine intervention.

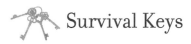 Survival Keys

* Don't always obey. Most people are taught that they should always respect and obey doctors, lawyers, and other authority figures. Unless that authority is heavenly, it is fallible.

* Believe your gut instincts. If your instincts prove wrong, the worst thing that can happen is people may laugh at you. Being laughed at will not kill you; being ignored very well might.

Chapter 43

MY FINAL CHAPTER, SWAN SONG, OR BOTH?

The best doctors in the world are
Doctor Diet, Doctor Quiet, and Doctor Merryman.
— Jonathan Swift (1667–1745)

♥ *Affirmation:* I choose love; I choose to heal.

Before leaving for my California vacation, I had serious questions about the inner voices that demanded I get an MRI, which I did. While basking in the warm California sun, I received no phone calls or emails from my doctors. I had circled my cell phone number in red ink when I filled out the paperwork and showed it to the admitting nurse so they couldn't miss it. Is no news good news? Were those voices and clowns just my imagination? I hope so!

The flight back from California is as uneventful as getting frisked by total strangers can be. It feels good to walk back into the familiarity of my Cape Cod kitchen. It's been almost five years to the day since I first started cancer treatment. How time flies. I cross the kitchen toward the family room to turn on the TV. A piece of torn notebook paper by the telephone catches my eye. It's a scribbled note dated three weeks earlier by our cat sitter. "Your doctors want you to call them about your test results." *Welcome home!* INCOMING!

The din in my brain is immediately replaced by my mother's frightened voice from years ago, "This disease is going to kill me!" Then,

Becky's voice replaces Mom's: "Why am I doing all these treatments when I know my cancer will come back and I'll be dead in five years?"

Five years, that magic number. My mind floods with voices of loved ones from the past and guides from the present. Will I hear voices in the future? Will I *have* a future or is this my swan song, too? Could I be lucky (or blessed) enough to survive cancer twice in one lifetime or am I hoping for too much? *Stop those negative thoughts!* I chide myself. *Maybe the doctors only want to tell you that your test results were fine and that you're healthy.* As if in response to my statement, the light on the message machine blinked ... RED!

The next morning, I arrive on my doctor's doorstep without an appointment. He whisks me into his examining room and closes the door behind us. "Kathy, we tried to call you, but your cat sitter said you were out of town."

"That's why I left my cell phone number circled in red on the MRI paperwork."

He continues, "We're all in a state of shock over your MRI results and have already held a meeting with all the hospital department heads." He looks into my eyes to see if that statement registered. It did. Bad news! The voices were not my imagination, and a meeting with the department heads doesn't surprise me. They are all my doctors anyway! It's obvious that the mad tea party isn't over yet. Time to move down to the next treatment again. These test results teach me Life Lesson #8: it's better to listen to my intuition and live with my own choices than to die from someone else's mistakes.

"According to the MRI, you have a five-centimeter tumor in your left breast, not the original right breast. It didn't show up on the mammograms. I know you asked for an MRI, but at that time it wasn't hospital policy to give them without a good reason," Dr. Harold says as I sit on the paper-covered examining table. I pick at my nail polish while he manipulates the area above my nipple. He shakes his head. He still can't feel anything out of the ordinary.

"This has happened twice to me in five years. Hospital policies have not been my friend because I am not 'the norm.'" Dr. Harold

nods, sits down in the chair across from me, and pens some notes
in my chart. This felt like an excellent moment to segue into voices,
spiritual guides, and angels, but since I didn't hear an inner voice say,
"*Yeah, tell him now!*" I decide to keep them to myself — especially
since I need these doctors again. Now that I finally have their undivided attention, what would I accomplish anyhow besides possibly
wigging them out?

All the same, here I am again, and only a few months shy of that
all-important five years cancer-free mark. Guess I didn't make it.
Unfortunately, my dream about the three crabs back in April makes
perfect sense. I think we found the third crab in my other breast, and
it's a real killer. I've definitely figured out the clowns.

Get a grip, I say to myself as I grip the table's edge. But I've learned
Life Lesson #9 from UHK. "Life isn't about holding your breath or
waiting for the storm to pass, because life is a procession of storms.
Life is about learning to sing in the wind and dance in the rain." That's
what makes life a sack of shit and giggles, so hold your nose and laugh
while you dance the dance of life — two steps forward, one step back.

"All hospitals have policies," Dr. Harold says and puts his pen in his
white coat pocket. "Is the fact that some women have false negative
mammograms, with no indication of cancer, before having a positive
MRI twice within five years reason enough to change a bad policy?" I
ask quietly but not unkindly. He nods and turns away.

I realize doctors are bound by policy, as are most big corporations,
but they took an oath to their patients, not the hospital. If they're
smart enough to be doctors, surely they're bright enough to find a
way around a bad policy and protect their patients. That old saying
"Wrong me once, shame on you; wrong me twice, shame on me," drifts
through my mind. I'm confused and angry, but do I only have myself
to blame? Some words of wisdom by Dr. Robert Anthony, an inspirational writer, pop into my mind: "When you blame others you give
up your power to change." I agree.

The blame game is a losing proposition. I must move beyond anger
and thoughts of being a victim. I'm not a bug on the windshield of
life, I am the windshield. All of this doesn't seem fair, but as I used

to tell my students, "Life isn't fair; it's real, so deal." "*Touché*," I whisper to myself. "Another past lesson to the rescue."

"I'm sorry. What did you say?" Dr. Harold asks.

"Nothing, just thinking out loud."

"Let's not jump the gun and assume this mass is cancer before we test to see if it's malignant or benign. I guess mammograms and blood tests are not your friends," he says, a hint of sadness in his voice.

I realize by his tone that it must be difficult for a doctor to watch a patient suffer a second time with a disease he thought was cured or at the very least in remission. I had appeared the picture of perfect health. Five years as doctor and patient has bonded us and made us different comrades in arms from the women in my chat group. I look past the forced smile and into the sad blue eyes devoid of their sparkle and respond, "True. But thank goodness MRIs are," then silently add *and my guides, too.*

Some people, especially the scientifically inclined, don't think outside the box well. From conversations with other scientists, and "regular" people for that matter, I've realized that outside the box can be considered a threat. It's outside their comfort zone. It's as though they fear some different infectious thought might invade them, like a computer virus, and destroy their perfect order. To explain how spiritual guides knew what doctors, mammograms, and blood tests didn't know, twice, might be too far outside the box for most scientists. Better that I keep this information to myself, lest they have me committed. But then, I could be completely wrong. I could simply be extremely lucky in catching cancer that medical tests missed twice in five years. That would be like winning the lottery twice in a row. What are the odds? Luck had little to do with this. Divine intervention did.

In a perfect world, I would say to Dr. Harold, "I knew about all this medical information that scientific equipment and tests missed because my spiritual voices and guides told me in meditations and dreams. They stood beside me when my mammogram was read, and they pointed to my right breast. That's why the mammography physician phoned you and said I seemed distressed." And my doctor would then throw his arms around me and cry, "Yes! Yes! I have those voices and guides, too. I'm so glad you shared this with me. Now I know you know, and you know I know." *Not!* I hear my guides laughing their heads off — and they don't laugh very often. I'll let the doctors read it in the book I've just decided to write. By then, I'll either be dead and it won't matter what anyone thinks, or I'll be healed and able to enlighten them to the fact that they were participants in a double-blind study between conventional medical tests and intuition — and the intuition won.

Honestly, I'm too busy to die. I have a book to write during a second course of cancer treatment while I keep more journals. I won't have time to fit in death. Death must wait again.

If only I'd known then what I know now. In a perfect world, when I approached Dr. Wagner five years ago with my first invisible lump, he would have responded with, "I don't feel anything, and you had a healthy mammogram, but let's take a look at the area with an ultrasound machine since I have one in the office. If we still don't see anything, I'll set up an appointment for an MRI. If something shows up on the MRI, we can do a needle biopsy and consult an oncologist." Yeah, in a perfect world. Now back to the real world.

Despite the hint of hope Dr. Harold holds for the biopsy results, I already know them. My guides would not have screamed in my ear and appeared in my dreams for something benign. My only hope is that it's not too late. A five-centimeter mass is stage-4 terminal. In my mind's eye, the caterpillar asks again, "Whooo are yooou?" while my reflection in the mirror asks, "How far down the rabbit hole do you want to go?" Have I finally hit bottom?

I wish I'd gotten that MRI sooner. But would it have mattered? Everything seems to have happened at the ideal time and in the right manner. It appears perfect in its imperfection. There's a strange order to this chaos. If going through this shit has saved one other life by changing useless hospital policies, then maybe it was worth it.

"Your needle biopsy is set for tomorrow, and we should have the results in a couple of days. Dr. Reddens is the best in her field. Is there anything else I can get for you now?" Dr. Harold asks as I calmly button my shirt.

"Yes, a pencil and paper. I want to write a book and start a second journal, right now."

"I want to read that book," Dr. Harold says, and turns to shut down the computer.

I think I just heard my guide chuckle. Will Dr. Harold hold another meeting for the department heads after he reads my book — especially the intuitive nightmare of the clowns? I'd love to be a fly on that wall. "I'll make sure you get a copy," I reply and slide off the table.

Now I know why I kept all those journals and didn't have that bonfire. I must find every scrap of paper I wrote on and compile the book I never intended to write in order to save my life a second time. My spiritual guides taught me two more important life lessons: #10 and #11: Be your own advocate; life is not a spectator sport, so roll up your sleeves and get dirty. Is this prophetic destiny, blind good luck, or Divine intervention? Today is a turning point. I could feel sorry for myself, angry at the world, or frozen with fear by memories. Knowledge is a double-edged sword. It robs the person of the "bliss of ignorance" and replaces it with lifesaving information. It's human to be in pain, but this time I chose not to suffer.

Life Lesson #12: Acknowledge your fears but don't let them rule your life. Combine them with the power of WORD. Reflecting on these past five years, I've found that life lessons come in groups. They're siblings related by challenges, yet uniquely different; Calamity's offspring, delivered by Dr. Crisis and baptized by Friar Fire.

On the way out of the hospital, a line has formed behind a bent-over elderly woman as she stands in the passage between the automatic doors. Her daughter pulls her arm in an effort to guide her over the threshold into modern medicine. Their bodies are reflected in the mirror-like doors, with my own superimposed reflection. I watch them watch me through refracted time, held between the glass microscope slides of life.

The woman tilts her head and apologetically declares, "I'm old." Then she takes a tiny step forward. I tell her that I think she's a winner. "Why?" she asks, and stops dead in her tracks. The doors flutter with curiosity and hold us in the narrow beams of their automatic eyes.

"The saying, 'He who dies with the most toys wins,' should be 'He who dies of old age with the most love wins,' because you can take love with you."

"I'm a winner then," she says, and holding tight to her daughter takes the final step.

I walk through the refracted reflections of my being and into the blinding light of an uncertain future, secure in the knowledge that no one walks alone and that self-advocating and questioning authority is healthy. Without it the world would still be flat. In the words of playwright Eugene Ionesco, "Ideology separates us. Dreams and anguish bring us together."

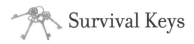 ## Survival Keys

* Welcome your learning steps. The Circle of Life is a series of learning steps taken through doors of experience.

* Crisis is part of life's hierarchy of order.

EPILOGUE

Readers are invited to join Kat's petition to include thermography among the medical technology choices in the detection and treatment of breast cancer and other cancers in women and men. You can sign the petition via www.accessyourinnerguide.com.

To purchase and download the guided meditations in this book, as well as other meditations in Kat's Health and Healing series, visit www.accessyourinnerguide.com/meditation-downloads/.

Kat has various sites and blogs dedicated to providing information to help those facing a health crisis. You can access these via the website www.survivingcancerland.com.

For more information on tapping into the power of your dreams, download Kat's free guidebook: *Access, Awaken and Your Inner Guide* via this link: www.accessyourinnerguide.com/workbook-link-page.

To review two pages of medical records that confirm the events this book describes regarding Kat's original and ultimate diagnoses, visit www.accessyourinnerguide.com/medical-records.

ADDITIONAL
MIND-BODY-HEALTH READING

Chopra, Deepak. *How to Know God: The Soul's Journey into the Mystery of Mysteries*. New York: Crown Publishers, 2000.

Hamilton, Allen J., M.D., FACS. *The Scalpel and the Soul*. New York: Jeremy P. Tarcher/Penguin, 2008.

Lipton, Bruce H., Ph.D. *The Biology of Belief*. Santa Rosa, CA: Mountain of Love/Elite Books, 2005.

Siegel, Bernie, M.D. *A Book of Miracles: Inspiring True Stores of Healing*. Novato, CA: New World Library, 2011.

Walden, Kelly Sullivan. *I Had the Strangest Dream ... The Dreamer's Dictionary for the 21st Century*. NY: Warner Books, 2006.

Wake Up Women: BE Happy, Healthy & Wealthy (Karen Mayfield, compiler). Global Partnership LLC, 2008.

Resources

Health and Testing

CSRA tests = Chemo Sensitivity and Resistance Assay
Rational Therapeutics, Long Beach, CA- 562 989-6455
www.rational-t.com/

Dr. Robert A. Nagourney, Medical Director, Memorial Medical
Center

Emotional and Financial Resources

R. A. Bloch Cancer Foundation Hotline 800 433-0464;
www.blochcancer.org
This organization provides phone counseling and mentors:
hotline@hrblock.com.

Diem Brown's foundation allows you to set up your own gift registry,
just like a wedding registry, during your crisis. Friends and family
can go online and purchase items from your "life list." Let them
know what you need, from kitchen gadgets to maid services and spa
treatments. Sign up at www.liveforthechallenge.com!

Resource sites that help women "bringin' home the bacon" with
advice on how to apply for disability: www.thedisabilityexpert.com/
and www.ssa.gov/applyfor disability/.

Rise Above It provides grants and scholarships for cancer survivors:
www.raibenefit.org.

Sites that can help with insurance and paperwork:
www.healthinsuranceinfo.net, www.patientadvocate.org, and
www.patient.cancerconsultants.com.

www.cancerpatienttravel.org offers charitable travel and housing arrangements, as does Sky Wish through Delta Airlines (800) UWA-2757, ext 285.

Enhance Your Book Club

Explore *Surviving Cancerland*'s numerous complexities that require differing viewpoints, such as:

Medical science vs. psychic intuition; and conventional therapy vs. holistic therapy.

Can these differences coexist and be complementary or only antagonistic?

Discuss which parts of the book you found to be the saddest and the most humorous.

Discuss ways in which people can self-advocate to avoid being victims of circumstance.

Dreams played a significant part in Kathy's diagnosis and her ability to self-advocate. How much importance do dreams have in your life? Would you believe them over medical science?

Discuss your feelings about spiritual guides, angels, inner voices, imaginary friends, and intuition. How are they alike or different? Does the idea of them impact your religious beliefs? How?

Give specific examples of how information in the book can help anyone in crisis.

Chapter 1
Dreams vs. Test, Again

The arrival of a good clown exercises a more
beneficial influence upon the health of a town than
the arrival of twenty asses laden with drugs.
— *Thomas Sydenham 1624–1689*

❧ *Affirmation:* I now have compassion,
even for those I do not understand. ❧

THE WORDS "LIFE COULD BE A DREAM — sh-boom" play on my radio alarm. Art mimicking life mimicking art. *Where does it stop,* I wonder as my morning dream evaporates. I was always a dreamer, but I never dreamed that I'd be a writer or recurrent cancer survivor. When I grew up, I wanted to be a Playboy bunny with gorgeous hair, a beautiful face, and perfect breasts. As a skinny girl of eight who was easily influenced by society's culture of sex and beauty, I was sure those breasts were what everyone wanted.

It's Saturday morning in Berlin, Germany, 1962. Branches from the Grunewald's trees that line KDV Boulevard scratch against my window-pane like the claws of a cat begging for shelter. Our apartment is cold and filled with the dampness of daybreak. No American tanks rumble down KDV to face the Russian tanks that line The Wall. The cold war takes the weekends off in Berlin.

I know what Mom will say if I creep into her room down the hall. "Kathy, please. Let us sleep until nine." A treat after night shifts nursing at Berlin's McNaire Army Hospital.

Weekend mornings could be lonely for an army brat only child, but they were also golden opportunities for exploration into forbidden regions of life that were considered too mature for proper little girls. I listen again for any sounds of movement.

Silence from the kitchen that housed Chippy the hamster tells of his surrender to sleep after another long night's attempt at freedom. His short-lived escapes always end in Dad's combat boots tucked beneath the wall radiator that heated my parents' bedroom. Their rhythmic breathing reassures me that no one will know.

With Gee-Gee, my imaginary childhood friend, by my side and my Barbie doll in my hand, I plop onto the hardwood floor beside the bed and slide a stolen *Playboy* magazine from under it — a prize pilfered from someone else and secretly traded for five comic books last Saturday morning. I cross my legs under me, opened the musty pages to the well-smudged centerfold, and gaze at her breasts in awe.

We're not alone anymore. We're in another place and time — my future.

I adjust my head as I rotate the page and gaze at the woman in all her glory. Gee-Gee gawks at her with the curiosity of a nine-year-old boy as I peer expectantly at adulthood. She is every bit as beautiful as Barbie, the most beautiful doll in the world. I shiver from excitement rather than cold as my heart beats louder in my ears. To me, this Playboy bunny is the emblem of organic beauty at its best. I'm hopeful, envious, and eager. In those stolen moments, I dream that someday I'll grow up and have beautiful breasts, too. At least that's the consensus of opinion this morning between Barbie, Gee-Gee, and me.

My childhood dreams faded with time before they could be shattered, twice, by cancer. Doctors missed my breast cancer both times, but my dreams and spiritual guides, one of whom, I believe, was Gee-Gee, did not. Surviving recurrence was a road filled with potholes and hairpin turns. Now, decades later, I write about all of it — the good, the bad, and the ugly.

About Kathleen

Kathleen O'Keefe-Kanavos, intuitive life and dream coach, survived three breast cancers that, missed by conventional medical tests, were diagnosed by her dreams. Kathleen chronicled her journey in dream journals, which she then used to write *Surviving Cancerland: Intuitive Aspects of Healing.* Kat taught special education in the Florida Lee County School System for ten years, working with profoundly disturbed and learning-disabled students, and taught psychology at the University of South Florida in Fort Myers. Kathleen is an R.A. Bloch Cancer Foundation Hotline phone counselor. She lives in Palm Beach, Cape Cod, and Rancho Mirage, California, with her husband of over thirty years and their three cats.

Speaking Experience

Drawing upon the wisdom she acquired from her medical odyssey, Kathleen has become a sought-after speaker, sharing her story via TV, radio, and at events such as telesummits, expos, international conferences, and support and association meetings, offering insight, advice, and comfort to cancer patients, survivors, and their loved ones, caregivers, and doctors.

Kathleen's Keynote Series includes:

* Access Your Inner Guidance Through Dreams, Prayers, and Meditations

* Dreams: Your Doorway to Better Health, Wealth, and Relationships

* Dreams: Answers to Your Voiced and Unvoiced Intentions

* Start Living Your Dream Life—Today!

Media Experience

Kathleen has been the subject of feature stories in many magazines and newspapers and is a featured blogger on sites such as the International Association for the Study of Dreams (IASD), DreamsCloud, Patheos, OMTimes Magazine, and Breast Cancer Yoga. She is a cancer and dream columnist for a number of online women's magazines, including CapeWomenOnline, and co-hosts, with Suzanne Strisower, the Living Well Talk Radio Network, including the Nautilus Book Awards Author Spotlight.

Details are available on Kathleen's websites:
SurvivingCancerland.com
and
AccessYourInnerGuide.com.

Contact Information

To schedule an interview or speaking engagement, contact:
Steve Allen Media
661 255-8283
media@steveallen.net

or

Mary Cate O'Malley
760 473-6545
marycate@omalleyconsulting.com